MW00888181

CONTENTS

CHAPTER 1: ANATOMY AND PHYSIOLOGY OF THE BLADDER

Introduction to Interstitial Cystitis/Bladder Pain Syndrome (IC/BPS)

Interstitial Cystitis/Bladder Pain Syndrome (IC/BPS) is a complex and multifaceted disorder characterized by chronic pelvic pain, pressure, or discomfort related to the bladder, often accompanied by urinary symptoms such as frequency and urgency. This condition presents a significant challenge for both patients and healthcare providers due to its variable presentation, the lack of a definitive diagnostic test, and the complexity of its management.

Definition and Clinical Manifestation

IC/BPS is defined by its hallmark symptoms: chronic pelvic pain and discomfort, often localized to the bladder and pelvic region, which can severely impact an individual's quality of life. The pain experienced by patients may range from a dull ache to severe discomfort and can be exacerbated by bladder filling or certain activities. In addition to pain, patients frequently report increased urinary frequency, urgency, and sometimes nocturia (nighttime urination). These symptoms can lead to significant disruptions in daily life, including difficulties with work, social activities, and overall emotional well-being.

Epidemiology

The prevalence of IC/BPS is estimated to affect between 3-6% of the population, with a higher incidence in women compared to men. The condition often emerges in individuals between the ages of 30 and 50, though it can occur in younger or older populations. The reasons for this gender disparity are not fully understood but may involve hormonal, anatomical, or psychosocial factors.

Pathophysiology and Etiology

The exact pathophysiology of IC/BPS remains elusive, making it a challenging condition to diagnose and treat effectively. Several theories have been proposed to explain the underlying mechanisms of IC/BPS:

1. **Urothelial Dysfunction:** One leading theory suggests that IC/BPS is associated with a defect in the bladder's urothelium, the lining of the bladder that acts as a barrier to harmful substances. Damage or dysfunction of the urothelium may lead to increased permeability, allowing irritating substances to reach the bladder wall and cause inflammation and pain.

2. **Inflammatory Response:** Chronic inflammation is thought to play a crucial role in IC/BPS. Some patients exhibit inflammatory changes in the bladder wall, including mast cell activation and the release of pro-inflammatory mediators, which can contribute to the sensation of pain.

3. **Autoimmune Mechanisms:** There is evidence suggesting that IC/BPS may involve an autoimmune component, where the body's immune system mistakenly targets its own tissues. This hypothesis is supported by the presence of other autoimmune conditions in some patients with IC/BPS.

4. **Neurogenic Factors:** Abnormalities in nerve pathways

and sensory processing may also contribute to IC/BPS. This includes heightened sensitivity of bladder nerves and altered pain processing in the central nervous system, which may amplify the perception of bladder pain.

5. **Infectious and Post-Infectious Models:** Some theories propose that IC/BPS may result from a previous urinary tract infection that leads to lasting changes in bladder function and pain sensitivity, even after the infection has resolved.

Diagnosis

Diagnosing IC/BPS is particularly challenging due to the absence of specific biomarkers or imaging findings and the overlap of symptoms with other urological and gynecological conditions. The diagnosis is typically based on a combination of clinical criteria, symptom history, and exclusion of other potential causes of similar symptoms.

Diagnostic criteria often include:

- Persistent pelvic pain for at least six months.
- Pain associated with bladder filling and relieved by urination.
- Exclusion of other conditions that could mimic IC/BPS symptoms, such as urinary tract infections, bladder cancer, and endometriosis.

A thorough evaluation usually involves a detailed patient history, physical examination, and various diagnostic tests, including urinalysis, urine culture, cystoscopy (bladder examination using a scope), and urodynamic studies to assess bladder function.

Management and Treatment

Management of IC/BPS is multimodal and tailored to the individual patient. Treatment strategies may include:

- **Pharmacological Approaches:** Medications to manage pain and inflammation, such as analgesics, anti-inflammatory drugs, and antidepressants. Bladder instillations with agents like dimethyl sulfoxide (DMSO) or heparin are also used to directly address bladder irritation.

- **Non-Pharmacological Therapies:** Physical therapy for pelvic floor dysfunction, dietary changes to avoid irritants, and behavioral therapies to manage pain and stress.

- **Interventional and Surgical Options:** For refractory cases, procedures such as bladder hydrodistention (stretching the bladder), neuromodulation (e.g., sacral nerve stimulation), and surgical options may be considered.

Impact on Quality of Life

The impact of IC/BPS on quality of life can be profound. The persistent nature of the symptoms often leads to significant emotional distress, including anxiety and depression. Patients may experience limitations in daily activities, disruptions in social and occupational roles, and a reduced overall quality of life.

Conclusion

Interstitial Cystitis/Bladder Pain Syndrome is a complex, chronic condition that requires a nuanced understanding and a comprehensive approach to diagnosis and treatment. Despite ongoing research, much remains to be learned about its etiology and optimal management strategies. Multidisciplinary care involving urologists, pain specialists, physical therapists, and mental health professionals is often necessary to provide holistic and effective treatment for patients suffering from IC/BPS. Continued research and clinical advancements are crucial to improving outcomes and enhancing the quality of life for individuals affected by this challenging condition.

Structure of the Bladder

The bladder is a crucial organ within the human urinary system, responsible for storing and expelling urine. Its structure is finely tuned to perform these functions efficiently, with its anatomy reflecting both its role in urine storage and its ability to accommodate varying volumes of liquid. This section delves into the detailed anatomy of the bladder, including its layers, internal features, and associated structures.

Anatomy and Overall Structure

The bladder is a hollow, muscular organ located in the pelvic cavity. It is shaped like a distensible sac and is positioned anterior to the rectum in males and the uterus in females. The bladder is primarily composed of smooth muscle tissue, connective tissue, and a specialized epithelial lining, all of which contribute to its functionality.

Layers of the Bladder Wall

The bladder wall is composed of several distinct layers, each playing a specific role in the bladder's overall function. These layers, from the innermost to the outermost, are:

1. **Mucosa (Urothelium):**
   - The mucosa is the innermost lining of the bladder, composed of transitional epithelium, also known as urothelium. This specialized epithelial tissue is unique to the urinary system and is designed to withstand the cyclic changes in bladder volume and pressure.
   - The urothelium consists of several layers of cells that are capable of stretching and contracting as the bladder fills and empties. The outermost cells of the urothelium are often dome-shaped when the bladder is full,

but flatten out as the bladder empties.

- Beneath the urothelium lies the lamina propria, a thin layer of connective tissue that supports the epithelial lining and contains blood vessels and nerves.

2. **Submucosa:**
   - The submucosa is a layer of connective tissue located beneath the lamina propria. It provides structural support to the bladder and contains additional blood vessels and nerve endings.
   - This layer is crucial for maintaining the integrity of the bladder wall and facilitating the blood supply required for bladder function.

3. **Muscularis (Detrusor Muscle):**
   - The muscularis, or detrusor muscle, is a thick layer of smooth muscle that constitutes the main muscular component of the bladder wall. It is responsible for bladder contraction during urination.
   - The detrusor muscle is organized into three interlacing layers: an inner longitudinal layer, a middle circular layer, and an outer longitudinal layer. This arrangement allows for efficient contraction and relaxation of the bladder during the storage and expulsion of urine.

4. **Adventitia (Serosa):**
   - The adventitia is the outermost layer of the bladder wall, consisting of connective tissue that helps anchor the bladder to surrounding structures. In the areas where the bladder is not covered by peritoneum, this layer is

known as the adventitia.

- In regions where the bladder is covered by peritoneum, such as the superior aspect, this layer is referred to as the serosa. The serosa provides a smooth surface that reduces friction between the bladder and adjacent structures.

Internal Features of the Bladder

Within the bladder's internal cavity, several important features and structures facilitate its function:

1. **Trigone:**
   - The trigone is a triangular area located at the base of the bladder, defined by the openings of the two ureters (which drain urine from the kidneys) and the internal urethral orifice (which leads to the urethra).
   - The trigone is a relatively smooth and non-distensible region compared to the rest of the bladder and plays a role in preventing the backflow of urine into the ureters.

2. **Bladder Neck:**
   - The bladder neck is the region where the bladder connects to the urethra. It is a crucial site for the regulation of urine flow and the prevention of involuntary leakage.
   - The internal urethral sphincter, comprised of smooth muscle fibers, is located at the bladder neck and helps control the release of urine.

3. **Rugae:**
   - Rugae are folds or ridges in the bladder wall that allow the organ to expand as it fills with urine. These folds are particularly prominent when the bladder is empty and gradually

smooth out as the bladder fills.

- The presence of rugae increases the surface area of the bladder and contributes to its ability to accommodate varying volumes of urine.

Blood Supply and Innervation

The blood supply to the bladder is primarily provided by the superior and inferior vesical arteries, which are branches of the internal iliac arteries. Venous blood is drained through the vesical venous plexus into the internal iliac veins.

The bladder is richly innervated by both the sympathetic and parasympathetic nervous systems:

- **Sympathetic Innervation:** The sympathetic fibers arise from the lumbar spinal cord and are involved in bladder relaxation and the control of the internal sphincter during urine storage.
- **Parasympathetic Innervation:** The parasympathetic fibers originate from the sacral spinal cord and are responsible for stimulating bladder contraction during urination.

Clinical Relevance

Understanding the structure of the bladder is crucial for diagnosing and managing various urological conditions. Disorders such as interstitial cystitis/bladder pain syndrome (IC/BPS), bladder cancer, and urinary tract infections can significantly impact the bladder's anatomy and function. Knowledge of the bladder's structure helps clinicians interpret diagnostic tests, plan appropriate treatments, and understand the pathophysiology of these conditions.

Conclusion

The bladder's structure is a testament to its complex and adaptive nature, designed to store and expel urine efficiently.

From its specialized urothelium to its robust muscular layers, every component plays a vital role in maintaining normal urinary function. A thorough understanding of bladder anatomy is essential for addressing bladder-related disorders and ensuring optimal patient care.

Urothelium and Its Functions

The urothelium, also known as transitional epithelium, is a specialized epithelial tissue that lines the bladder, ureters, and part of the urethra. This unique epithelial layer plays a crucial role in the urinary system, serving both protective and functional purposes. Understanding the structure and function of the urothelium is essential for comprehending how the bladder operates and how various conditions, such as Interstitial Cystitis/Bladder Pain Syndrome (IC/BPS), affect bladder function.

Structure of the Urothelium

The urothelium is a type of stratified epithelium composed of several layers of cells, each contributing to the tissue's unique properties:

1. **Cell Layers:**
   - **Surface Layer (Umbrella Cells):** The outermost layer of the urothelium consists of large, dome-shaped cells known as umbrella cells. These cells are adapted to handle the stretch and pressure changes that occur as the bladder fills and empties. The umbrella cells have a unique morphology that allows them to flatten when the bladder is distended and revert to a more dome-shaped appearance when the bladder is empty.
   - **Intermediate Layers:** Beneath the umbrella cells are several layers of intermediate cells.

These cells are polygonal and less specialized than the umbrella cells but still contribute to the bladder's ability to stretch and accommodate changes in volume.

- **Basal Layer:** The innermost layer consists of basal cells, which are smaller, cuboidal cells that act as a reservoir for cell regeneration. Basal cells can differentiate into intermediate and umbrella cells as needed to repair and replenish the urothelium.

2. **Cell Junctions and Barrier Function:**
    - The urothelium is characterized by tight junctions between its cells, which create a barrier that prevents the leakage of urine and protects underlying tissues from harmful substances. These tight junctions are crucial for maintaining the integrity of the urothelial lining and preventing urine from causing irritation or damage to the bladder wall.

Functions of the Urothelium

The urothelium performs several critical functions that are integral to the proper functioning of the urinary system:

1. **Barrier Function:**
    - The primary function of the urothelium is to act as a selective barrier between the urine and the underlying tissues of the bladder. This barrier prevents the diffusion of potentially toxic substances present in urine into the bladder wall and the bloodstream. The tight junctions between urothelial cells are essential for maintaining this barrier function and protecting the bladder from damage.

2. **Protective Function:**

- The urothelium is equipped with various protective mechanisms that shield it from the harsh environment of the bladder. It secretes a protective layer of glycosaminoglycans (GAGs) and other mucopolysaccharides onto its surface. This layer helps to neutralize the effects of urine and reduces the friction between the bladder wall and the urine.

3. **Storage and Stretching:**
   - One of the most remarkable features of the urothelium is its ability to accommodate significant changes in bladder volume. As the bladder fills with urine, the urothelium stretches and becomes thinner. The umbrella cells play a key role in this stretching ability by flattening out and increasing their surface area. When the bladder empties, the urothelium returns to its original, more layered configuration.

4. **Sensory Function:**
   - The urothelium also has sensory functions. It contains specialized sensory receptors that detect changes in bladder volume and the presence of irritating substances in the urine. These sensory signals are transmitted to the nervous system, helping regulate bladder function and prompting the sensation of urgency and the need to void.

5. **Regenerative Capacity:**
   - The urothelium possesses a high regenerative capacity, which is crucial for maintaining its integrity and function over time. The basal cells at the innermost layer can rapidly proliferate and differentiate into intermediate and umbrella cells to repair any damage

or loss of urothelial cells. This regenerative ability is vital for recovering from injury or stress, such as that caused by infections or mechanical trauma.

Role in Disease and Dysfunction

When the urothelium is compromised or dysfunctional, it can lead to various pathological conditions. For example:

1. **Interstitial Cystitis/Bladder Pain Syndrome (IC/BPS):**
   - In IC/BPS, the urothelium is often damaged or dysfunctional. Studies have shown that patients with IC/BPS may have a defective urothelial barrier, which allows irritating substances in the urine to contact the bladder wall and trigger inflammation and pain. The integrity of the urothelial lining is crucial for preventing these adverse effects.

2. **Bladder Cancer:**
   - The urothelium is the tissue from which most bladder cancers arise. Changes in urothelial cells, such as dysplasia or neoplasia, can lead to malignant transformations. Understanding the normal structure and function of the urothelium is important for recognizing abnormal changes that may indicate cancer.

3. **Urinary Tract Infections (UTIs):**
   - The urothelium plays a role in defending against infections. Damage to the urothelial lining can increase susceptibility to UTIs, as the protective barrier is weakened, allowing pathogens to penetrate more easily.

Current Research and Future Directions

Ongoing research into the urothelium focuses on understanding its role in various diseases and developing targeted therapies. Advances in cellular and molecular biology have provided deeper insights into urothelial cell function, signaling pathways, and regenerative mechanisms. Emerging therapies aim to restore or enhance urothelial function, such as by using growth factors or regenerative medicine techniques to repair damaged urothelium.

Conclusion

The urothelium is a highly specialized and functional epithelial tissue that plays essential roles in the urinary system. Its ability to act as a barrier, protect underlying tissues, accommodate bladder stretching, sense changes, and regenerate makes it integral to normal bladder function. Understanding the structure and functions of the urothelium is crucial for diagnosing and treating conditions that affect the bladder and urinary tract, highlighting the importance of continued research and clinical investigation in this area.

Bladder Musculature: Detrusor and Sphincters

The bladder is a highly specialized organ whose primary functions include storing and expelling urine. The efficient performance of these functions depends significantly on its musculature, particularly the detrusor muscle and the sphincters. Understanding the structure, function, and coordination of these muscular components is crucial for grasping how the bladder operates and how various disorders may impact its function.

Detrusor Muscle

The detrusor muscle is the primary muscular component of the bladder wall and plays a central role in the storage and expulsion of urine. Its structure and function are integral to the bladder's ability to accommodate varying volumes of urine and to contract effectively during micturition (urination).

1. **Anatomy and Structure:**
   - **Composition:** The detrusor muscle is composed of smooth muscle fibers arranged in three interlacing layers: an inner longitudinal layer, a middle circular layer, and an outer longitudinal layer. This multi-layered arrangement allows for coordinated contraction and relaxation of the bladder.

   - **Smooth Muscle Fibers:** Unlike skeletal muscle, which is under voluntary control, the smooth muscle fibers of the detrusor muscle are involuntary and controlled by the autonomic nervous system. These fibers are elongated and spindle-shaped, connected by gap junctions that facilitate coordinated contractions.

2. **Function:**
   - **Urine Storage:** During the storage phase, the detrusor muscle remains relaxed to accommodate the increasing volume of urine. This relaxation is facilitated by sympathetic nervous system activity, which inhibits detrusor contractions and prevents involuntary voiding.

   - **Urination (Micturition):** During urination, the detrusor muscle contracts in a coordinated manner to expel urine from the bladder. This contraction is primarily controlled by parasympathetic nervous system activity, which stimulates the detrusor muscle to contract while simultaneously relaxing the internal sphincter.

3. **Innervation and Control:**

- **Sympathetic Nervous System:** The sympathetic nerves (primarily the hypogastric nerve) release norepinephrine, which inhibits detrusor contractions and maintains bladder relaxation during the storage phase.

- **Parasympathetic Nervous System:** The parasympathetic nerves (via the pelvic nerve) release acetylcholine, which stimulates detrusor contraction during the micturition phase. The balance between sympathetic and parasympathetic activity ensures proper bladder function.

4. **Clinical Relevance:**
   - **Overactive Bladder:** Conditions like overactive bladder (OAB) are characterized by excessive and involuntary detrusor contractions, leading to symptoms such as urinary urgency and frequency.

   - **Detrusor Instability:** In detrusor instability or detrusor overactivity, inappropriate or uncoordinated contractions can lead to leakage or urinary incontinence.

Sphincters of the Bladder

The sphincters are crucial for controlling the flow of urine from the bladder through the urethra. They consist of two main components: the internal urethral sphincter and the external urethral sphincter. Each plays a distinct role in maintaining urinary continence and coordinating micturition.

1. **Internal Urethral Sphincter:**
   - **Anatomy and Structure:** The internal urethral sphincter is composed of smooth muscle fibers and is located at the junction between the bladder and the urethra. It

encircles the bladder neck and acts as an involuntary control mechanism.

- ◦ **Function:** The internal sphincter maintains tonic contraction to prevent involuntary leakage of urine during the storage phase. During micturition, the parasympathetic nervous system induces relaxation of the internal sphincter, allowing urine to pass into the urethra.

- ◦ **Clinical Relevance:** Dysfunction of the internal sphincter can contribute to urinary incontinence and may be involved in conditions such as bladder outlet obstruction.

2. **External Urethral Sphincter:**
   - ◦ **Anatomy and Structure:** The external urethral sphincter is composed of striated skeletal muscle and is located around the distal part of the urethra. Unlike the internal sphincter, it is under voluntary control.

   - ◦ **Function:** The external sphincter provides voluntary control over the release of urine. It allows an individual to consciously initiate or delay urination. During the storage phase, the external sphincter is contracted to maintain continence. During micturition, it relaxes to allow urine flow.

   - ◦ **Clinical Relevance:** Damage or dysfunction of the external sphincter can lead to difficulties in controlling urination, resulting in stress urinary incontinence. Conditions such as pelvic floor dysfunction or neurological disorders can affect the external sphincter's function.

Coordination of Musculature

The coordination between the detrusor muscle and the sphincters is essential for normal bladder function. The process of micturition involves a complex interplay between these muscles:

1. **Storage Phase:**
   - During urine storage, the detrusor muscle remains relaxed due to sympathetic stimulation, and the internal and external sphincters are contracted to maintain continence. This coordination prevents involuntary leakage and allows the bladder to expand as it fills with urine.

2. **Micturition Phase:**
   - When micturition is initiated, the detrusor muscle contracts under parasympathetic stimulation, while the internal sphincter relaxes to permit urine flow into the urethra. The external sphincter voluntarily relaxes to allow the passage of urine. This process requires coordinated signals from the central nervous system to ensure that the detrusor muscle contracts efficiently and the sphincters relax appropriately.

Clinical Considerations and Disorders

Several conditions can disrupt the normal function of the bladder musculature, leading to various urinary symptoms:

1. **Detrusor Overactivity:** Characterized by involuntary contractions of the detrusor muscle, leading to symptoms such as urinary urgency, frequency, and incontinence. It may be associated with conditions like overactive bladder syndrome.

2. **Bladder Outlet Obstruction:** Conditions such as benign prostatic hyperplasia (BPH) or urethral stricture can obstruct the outlet of the bladder, leading

to increased detrusor pressure and difficulty in urine flow.

3. **Neurogenic Bladder:** Neurological disorders such as spinal cord injury or multiple sclerosis can disrupt the normal coordination between the detrusor muscle and sphincters, resulting in impaired bladder function.

4. **Stress Incontinence:** Involves the external sphincter and is characterized by involuntary leakage of urine during activities that increase abdominal pressure, such as coughing or exercise.

Conclusion

The bladder's musculature, comprising the detrusor muscle and sphincters, is essential for the proper storage and expulsion of urine. The detrusor muscle's coordinated contractions allow the bladder to accommodate varying volumes and expel urine efficiently, while the sphincters regulate the release of urine and maintain continence. Understanding the structure and function of these muscular components is critical for diagnosing and managing various bladder disorders and ensuring effective treatment strategies.

Nervous System Control of the Bladder

The bladder's complex function of storing and expelling urine is intricately regulated by the nervous system. This regulation involves a sophisticated network of neural pathways that coordinate both voluntary and involuntary aspects of bladder control. The nervous system control of the bladder encompasses sensory input, reflexive responses, and higher cognitive control, all of which work in concert to manage urinary function effectively. This section provides a detailed examination of the neural mechanisms underlying bladder control, including the roles of sympathetic and parasympathetic systems, spinal cord reflexes, and cortical influences.

Overview of Nervous System Control

The bladder's function is controlled by both autonomic (involuntary) and somatic (voluntary) nervous systems. This control involves:

- **Autonomic Nervous System (ANS):** Regulates the involuntary functions of the bladder, including smooth muscle contraction and relaxation.

- **Somatic Nervous System:** Provides voluntary control over the external urethral sphincter, allowing conscious regulation of urination.

Sympathetic Nervous System

1. **Anatomy and Pathways:**
   - The sympathetic nervous system (SNS) originates from the thoracolumbar region of the spinal cord (T11-L2). Sympathetic fibers travel through the hypogastric nerve to reach the bladder.

   - The sympathetic postganglionic fibers release norepinephrine, which acts on beta-adrenergic receptors to influence bladder function.

2. **Function:**
   - **Bladder Relaxation:** During the storage phase, sympathetic stimulation promotes relaxation of the detrusor muscle. This relaxation is achieved through beta-adrenergic receptor activation, which reduces detrusor muscle tone and increases bladder capacity.

   - **Internal Sphincter Contraction:** Simultaneously, the sympathetic nervous system maintains tonic contraction of the internal urethral sphincter, preventing involuntary leakage of urine.

3. **Clinical Relevance:**
    - **Overactive Bladder (OAB):** Conditions like OAB can involve dysregulation of sympathetic control, resulting in excessive bladder contractions and urinary urgency.
    - **Bladder Outlet Obstruction:** Conditions such as benign prostatic hyperplasia (BPH) can affect sympathetic control, leading to increased detrusor pressure and difficulty with bladder emptying.

Parasympathetic Nervous System

1. **Anatomy and Pathways:**
    - The parasympathetic nervous system (PNS) originates from the sacral spinal cord segments S2-S4. Parasympathetic fibers travel through the pelvic nerve to reach the bladder.
    - The postganglionic fibers release acetylcholine, which acts on muscarinic receptors to influence bladder function.

2. **Function:**
    - **Bladder Contraction:** During the micturition phase, parasympathetic stimulation facilitates contraction of the detrusor muscle. This contraction is mediated by muscarinic receptors (primarily M3 receptors), which increase bladder muscle tone and pressure, leading to the expulsion of urine.
    - **Internal Sphincter Relaxation:** The parasympathetic nervous system induces relaxation of the internal urethral sphincter, allowing urine to flow into the urethra.

3. **Clinical Relevance:**

- **Detrusor Overactivity:** In conditions like detrusor overactivity, there is excessive parasympathetic activity leading to frequent and urgent urination.
- **Neurogenic Bladder:** Damage to the parasympathetic pathways can result in impaired bladder contraction and incomplete emptying.

Spinal Cord Reflexes

1. **Micturition Reflex:**
   - **Mechanism:** The micturition reflex is a spinal reflex that initiates the process of urination. Stretch receptors in the bladder wall detect the filling of the bladder and send afferent signals to the spinal cord.
   - **Integration:** The spinal cord integrates these sensory signals and sends efferent signals through the parasympathetic nervous system to the detrusor muscle to contract and the internal sphincter to relax.
   - **Voluntary Modulation:** Higher brain centers can modulate this reflex. The reflex is typically under voluntary control, allowing individuals to delay urination until an appropriate time.

2. **Clinical Relevance:**
   - **Spinal Cord Injury:** Injuries to the spinal cord can disrupt the micturition reflex, leading to loss of bladder control, incontinence, or difficulties with bladder emptying depending on the level and severity of the injury.

Cortical and Supraspinal Control

1. **Role of the Brain:**

- **Cerebral Cortex:** The cerebral cortex, particularly the prefrontal cortex and parietal lobes, plays a critical role in the conscious control of micturition. It helps in deciding when and where to void, integrating sensory information with social and environmental cues.

- **Pontine Micturition Center:** The pontine micturition center, located in the brainstem, coordinates the timing of bladder contractions and sphincter relaxation. It acts as a relay between the spinal reflexes and higher cortical control.

2. **Clinical Relevance:**

   - **Neurological Disorders:** Conditions such as stroke, multiple sclerosis, and traumatic brain injury can affect cortical and pontine control of bladder function, leading to a range of symptoms from incontinence to urinary retention.

   - **Psychological Factors:** Stress and anxiety can also impact bladder function, highlighting the role of higher brain centers in modulating urinary control.

Integration and Coordination

1. **Coordination of Bladder Function:**

   - The bladder's function relies on the seamless integration of sympathetic, parasympathetic, and voluntary control mechanisms. Proper coordination ensures that the bladder can store urine efficiently and expel it at appropriate times.

   - The complex interaction between autonomic control (sympathetic and parasympathetic), spinal reflexes, and cortical input allows for both involuntary and voluntary regulation of bladder function.

2. **Clinical Considerations:**

    ◦ **Dysregulation:** Disorders of bladder control often involve dysregulation at multiple levels of this integrated system. For instance, conditions like overactive bladder may involve excessive parasympathetic activity, while stress urinary incontinence may result from impaired external sphincter control.

    ◦ **Management:** Effective management of bladder disorders often requires a multidisciplinary approach, including pharmacological interventions to modulate autonomic activity, physical therapy to strengthen pelvic muscles, and behavioral therapies to address cognitive and emotional factors.

Conclusion

The nervous system's control of the bladder is a complex and finely tuned process involving sympathetic and parasympathetic pathways, spinal reflexes, and higher cortical centers. This intricate network ensures that the bladder can efficiently store and expel urine while maintaining continence. Understanding the detailed mechanisms of bladder control is crucial for diagnosing and treating urinary disorders, as disruptions at any level of this system can lead to significant functional impairments. Continued research into the neurophysiology of bladder control promises to enhance our ability to manage and treat bladder-related conditions effectively.

Blood Supply and Lymphatic Drainage

The bladder, a vital organ in the urinary system, relies on a well-established network of blood vessels and lymphatic channels to maintain its function and overall health. The blood supply and lymphatic drainage are critical for delivering nutrients, removing waste products, and regulating bladder function. This section explores the anatomy and physiology of the bladder's blood supply and lymphatic drainage, emphasizing their roles in health and disease.

Blood Supply

The blood supply to the bladder is provided by a network of arteries that ensure adequate oxygenation and nutrient delivery to the bladder tissues. The primary sources of blood supply are the superior and inferior vesical arteries, which are branches of the internal iliac arteries.

1. **Superior Vesical Artery:**
   - **Origin:** The superior vesical artery originates from the umbilical artery, a branch of the internal iliac artery. In adults, it is typically a continuation of the umbilical artery after birth.
   - **Distribution:** It supplies blood to the upper portion of the bladder and the dome, as well as the adjacent parts of the ureter.
   - **Function:** The superior vesical artery provides essential oxygen and nutrients to the upper bladder wall, contributing to the maintenance of its normal function.

2. **Inferior Vesical Artery:**
   - **Origin:** The inferior vesical artery originates from the internal iliac artery. In females, this

artery may also be referred to as the vaginal artery when it supplies the vaginal wall.

- **Distribution:** It supplies blood to the lower portion of the bladder, including the bladder neck and the prostatic urethra in males or the anterior vaginal wall in females.

- **Function:** This artery ensures that the lower bladder wall and the surrounding structures receive adequate blood flow, which is crucial for maintaining the health of these tissues.

3. **Additional Vessels:**
   - **Obliterated Umbilical Artery:** In some cases, the obliterated umbilical artery, a remnant of fetal circulation, may contribute to the blood supply of the bladder.

   - **Branches of the Internal Pudendal Artery:** These branches may also supply blood to the bladder, particularly the posterior aspect and the base.

4. **Venous Drainage:**
   - The venous blood from the bladder is drained by the vesical venous plexus, which surrounds the bladder and drains into the internal iliac veins. The venous plexus is an intricate network of veins that parallels the arterial supply and collects deoxygenated blood from the bladder wall.

   - **Clinical Relevance:** Disruption of blood supply or venous drainage can lead to conditions such as ischemia, impaired bladder function, or complications following surgery. For instance, tumors or trauma may impact the vascular supply and require careful surgical planning.

Lymphatic Drainage

The lymphatic system plays a crucial role in maintaining fluid balance, removing interstitial fluid, and facilitating immune responses. The lymphatic drainage of the bladder ensures that excess fluid and waste products are efficiently removed, and it also plays a role in the metastatic spread of malignancies.

1. **Lymphatic Vessels:**
   - **Location:** Lymphatic vessels drain the bladder through a network of channels that accompany the blood vessels. These vessels follow the arterial and venous pathways, eventually converging into larger lymphatic trunks.

   - **Function:** The lymphatic vessels transport lymph, a clear fluid containing proteins, lipids, and immune cells, from the bladder wall to regional lymph nodes. This process helps in the removal of excess fluid and cellular debris and supports the immune response.

2. **Lymph Nodes:**
   - **External Iliac Nodes:** Lymphatic drainage from the bladder primarily flows into the external iliac lymph nodes. These nodes are located along the external iliac artery and are responsible for filtering lymph from the bladder and surrounding structures.

   - **Internal Iliac Nodes:** Some lymphatic vessels also drain into the internal iliac lymph nodes, which are situated near the internal iliac artery and contribute to the drainage of the lower pelvic structures.

   - **Sacral Nodes:** In certain cases, lymphatic drainage may reach the sacral lymph nodes located in the sacral region of the pelvis.

3. **Clinical Relevance:**
    - **Bladder Cancer:** The lymphatic drainage system is particularly important in the context of malignancies such as bladder cancer. Tumor cells can spread to regional lymph nodes, making them key sites for staging and treatment planning. Understanding the patterns of lymphatic drainage helps in assessing the extent of disease and planning appropriate interventions.

    - **Inflammatory Conditions:** Conditions such as chronic cystitis or interstitial cystitis may involve inflammatory responses that affect lymphatic drainage, potentially leading to localized edema or changes in lymphatic flow.

4. **Surgical Considerations:**
    - **Lymphadenectomy:** During bladder surgeries, particularly those involving cancer treatment, lymphadenectomy (removal of lymph nodes) may be performed to assess and manage the spread of disease. Knowledge of the lymphatic drainage pathways is essential for effectively targeting affected lymph nodes and minimizing the risk of recurrence.

Interaction Between Blood Supply and Lymphatic Drainage

The interplay between the blood supply and lymphatic drainage is crucial for maintaining bladder health. The blood supply ensures that the bladder receives adequate oxygen and nutrients, while the lymphatic system helps to remove waste products and regulate fluid balance. Disruptions in either system can impact bladder function and contribute to various clinical conditions.

1. **Fluid Balance:** Adequate blood flow supports the health of bladder tissues, while efficient lymphatic drainage helps manage interstitial fluid levels. Imbalances in fluid regulation can lead to symptoms such as edema or impaired bladder function.

2. **Tissue Repair and Response:** The blood supply provides essential components for tissue repair and immune responses, while lymphatic drainage helps clear cellular debris and inflammatory mediators. Effective collaboration between these systems is necessary for proper healing and recovery from injury or infection.

Summary

The bladder's blood supply and lymphatic drainage are essential components of its overall function and health. The arterial supply, primarily from the superior and inferior vesical arteries, ensures that the bladder receives adequate oxygen and nutrients. The venous drainage, through the vesical venous plexus, facilitates the removal of deoxygenated blood. The lymphatic system, including lymphatic vessels and nodes, plays a key role in fluid regulation, immune responses, and the spread of malignancies.

Understanding these systems is crucial for diagnosing and managing bladder-related conditions, including cancers, inflammatory diseases, and surgical complications. Advances in medical knowledge and technology continue to enhance our ability to address disorders affecting the bladder's vascular and lymphatic systems, ultimately improving patient outcomes and quality of life.

CHAPTER 2:
BIOCHEMISTRY AND
MOLECULAR BIOLOGY

Urothelial Barrier Function and Dysfunction

The urothelium, a specialized epithelial lining of the bladder, plays a critical role in maintaining the integrity and functionality of the urinary tract. This epithelial layer is not merely a passive barrier but an active participant in bladder homeostasis, protecting underlying tissues from the potentially harmful effects of urine and contributing to the regulation of bladder function. Understanding the urothelial barrier function and the mechanisms leading to its dysfunction is essential for comprehending various bladder disorders, including Interstitial Cystitis/Bladder Pain Syndrome (IC/BPS) and other conditions affecting bladder health.

Structure and Function of the Urothelial Barrier

The urothelium is a stratified epithelial tissue composed of several layers of cells, each contributing to the overall barrier function:

1. **Cell Layers:**
   - **Umbrella Cells:** The outermost layer of the urothelium consists of large, dome-shaped umbrella cells. These cells are adapted to withstand the mechanical stresses of bladder filling and emptying. Their unique morphology allows them to flatten out as the

bladder fills and return to a more dome-like shape as it empties.

- ◦ **Intermediate Cells:** Beneath the umbrella cells are several layers of intermediate cells. These cells are polygonal and contribute to the structural integrity and elasticity of the urothelium.

- ◦ **Basal Cells:** The innermost layer is made up of basal cells, which are smaller and cuboidal. These cells serve as progenitors for the regeneration of the urothelium.

2. **Barrier Function:**
   - ◦ **Tight Junctions:** The urothelium is characterized by tight junctions between its cells. These junctions form a selective barrier that prevents the leakage of urine into the underlying tissues and protects the bladder wall from potential irritants.

   - ◦ **Glycosaminoglycan (GAG) Layer:** On the apical surface of the urothelium, a layer of glycosaminoglycans (GAGs) and other mucopolysaccharides forms a protective coating. This layer helps to neutralize the potentially harmful effects of urine and reduce friction between the bladder wall and the urine.

3. **Sensory and Regulatory Functions:**
   - ◦ **Sensory Receptors:** The urothelium contains sensory receptors that detect changes in bladder volume and the presence of irritating substances. These receptors help regulate bladder function and trigger the sensation of urgency when needed.

   - ◦ **Regulatory Role:** The urothelium

releases various signaling molecules that influence bladder function, including neurotransmitters and growth factors that modulate inflammation, pain, and cellular repair.

Mechanisms of Urothelial Barrier Dysfunction

Urothelial barrier dysfunction can result from various factors, leading to impaired bladder function and contributing to the development of bladder disorders:

1. **Inflammation and Infection:**
   - **Chronic Inflammation:** Conditions such as chronic cystitis can lead to persistent inflammation of the urothelium, causing damage to the barrier. Inflammatory cytokines and immune cells can disrupt tight junctions and compromise barrier integrity.

   - **Infections:** Urinary tract infections (UTIs) can damage the urothelium, allowing bacteria and toxins to penetrate the bladder wall. Recurrent infections can exacerbate urothelial dysfunction and contribute to long-term damage.

2. **Mechanical Stress and Injury:**
   - **Bladder Overdistension:** Prolonged or repeated bladder overdistension, such as from chronic retention or high-pressure voiding, can damage the urothelium. This mechanical stress can lead to disruption of tight junctions and damage to the protective GAG layer.

   - **Trauma:** Physical trauma to the bladder, including surgical procedures or injury, can compromise the urothelial barrier and impair its ability to protect underlying tissues.

3. **Chemical and Environmental Factors:**
   ◦ **Irritants:** Exposure to chemical irritants, such as those found in certain medications or environmental toxins, can damage the urothelium. This damage can lead to disruption of the barrier and contribute to symptoms such as pain and urgency.
   ◦ **Dietary Factors:** Certain dietary components, such as acidic or spicy foods, can exacerbate bladder irritation and contribute to urothelial dysfunction in susceptible individuals.

4. **Genetic and Autoimmune Factors:**
   ◦ **Genetic Predisposition:** Genetic factors may predispose individuals to urothelial dysfunction. Variations in genes involved in urothelial cell function and repair can influence susceptibility to bladder disorders.
   ◦ **Autoimmune Responses:** Autoimmune conditions, such as interstitial cystitis/ bladder pain syndrome (IC/BPS), may involve immune-mediated damage to the urothelium. Autoantibodies and immune cells can target urothelial cells, leading to inflammation and barrier dysfunction.

Clinical Implications of Urothelial Dysfunction

Urothelial barrier dysfunction is associated with several clinical conditions and can have significant implications for patient health:

1. **Interstitial Cystitis/Bladder Pain Syndrome (IC/BPS):**
   ◦ **Pathophysiology:** IC/BPS is characterized by chronic bladder pain, increased urinary frequency, and urgency. Dysfunction of the urothelial barrier is thought to play a central role in this condition, as it allows irritating

substances in the urine to contact the bladder wall and trigger inflammation and pain.

- **Treatment Approaches:** Treatments for IC/BPS often focus on restoring urothelial barrier function and reducing inflammation. This may include medications that protect the bladder lining, such as oral pentosan polysulfate, and treatments aimed at reducing bladder irritation.

2. **Bladder Cancer:**
   - **Risk Factors:** Damage to the urothelium and persistent irritation are known risk factors for the development of bladder cancer. Chronic exposure to carcinogens or repeated irritation can lead to genetic mutations and dysplasia in urothelial cells.

   - **Management:** Early detection and treatment of bladder cancer often involve assessing the extent of urothelial damage and employing strategies to minimize further injury.

3. **Urinary Tract Infections (UTIs):**
   - **Impact on Barrier Function:** UTIs can cause acute damage to the urothelium, leading to symptoms such as pain and discomfort. Recurrent infections may contribute to long-term urothelial dysfunction and increased susceptibility to future infections.

   - **Preventive Measures:** Strategies to prevent UTIs and manage urothelial health include maintaining proper hygiene, avoiding irritants, and addressing any underlying conditions that may contribute to infection risk.

4. **Bladder Pain and Urgency:**

- **Symptoms:** Dysregulation of the urothelial barrier can lead to symptoms such as bladder pain, urgency, and frequent urination. These symptoms can significantly impact quality of life and may require comprehensive management approaches.

Diagnostic and Therapeutic Approaches

1. **Diagnostic Tools:**
   - **Cystoscopy:** Direct visualization of the bladder using cystoscopy can help assess the condition of the urothelium and identify any abnormalities or damage.
   - **Biopsy and Histology:** Biopsy of the bladder wall and histological examination can provide information on urothelial integrity, inflammation, and cellular changes.

2. **Therapeutic Strategies:**
   - **Medications:** Treatments aimed at restoring urothelial barrier function include medications that protect the bladder lining or reduce inflammation. Examples include oral pentosan polysulfate and intravesical treatments with agents like hyaluronic acid.
   - **Lifestyle Modifications:** Dietary changes and avoidance of known irritants can help manage symptoms and protect urothelial health.
   - **Physical Therapy:** Pelvic floor physical therapy can address issues related to bladder function and improve overall urinary health.

Conclusion

The urothelial barrier plays a crucial role in protecting the bladder from potentially harmful substances and maintaining its overall function. Dysfunction of this barrier can lead to a range of clinical conditions, including IC/BPS, UTIs, and bladder cancer. Understanding the mechanisms underlying urothelial barrier function and dysfunction is essential for diagnosing and managing these conditions effectively. Advances in research and treatment approaches continue to improve our ability to address bladder disorders and enhance patient outcomes.

Cellular and Molecular Mechanisms in Interstitial Cystitis/ Bladder Pain Syndrome (IC/BPS)

Interstitial Cystitis/Bladder Pain Syndrome (IC/BPS) is a chronic bladder condition characterized by pelvic pain, urinary frequency, and urgency, often without an identifiable infection or other clear etiology. The pathophysiology of IC/BPS is complex, involving a range of cellular and molecular mechanisms that disrupt normal bladder function and contribute to the symptoms experienced by patients. This section delves into the key cellular and molecular mechanisms implicated in IC/BPS, highlighting the roles of urothelial dysfunction, inflammatory responses, neurogenic factors, and changes in bladder tissue structure.

1. Urothelial Dysfunction

The urothelium, the bladder's protective epithelial lining, plays a crucial role in maintaining bladder health and function. Dysfunction of the urothelium is central to the pathogenesis of IC/BPS.

1. **Barrier Disruption:**
   ◦ **Glycosaminoglycan (GAG) Layer Deficiency:** The GAG layer on the surface of urothelial cells acts as a protective barrier against the potentially irritating substances in urine. In IC/BPS, there is often a reduction or dysfunction of this GAG

layer, leading to increased permeability and exposure of underlying tissues to harmful urinary constituents. This disruption can result in increased bladder irritation and inflammation.

- **Tight Junctions:** Tight junctions between urothelial cells maintain the barrier function of the urothelium. In IC/BPS, these junctions can be compromised, allowing for leakage of substances and contributing to the inflammatory response.

2. **Urothelial Cell Changes:**
   - **Cellular Injury:** The urothelium in IC/BPS may show signs of cellular injury, including apoptosis (programmed cell death) and increased turnover of urothelial cells. Damaged cells can contribute to a loss of barrier function and exacerbate symptoms.
   - **Altered Gene Expression:** Urothelial cells in IC/BPS may exhibit altered gene expression profiles, including changes in genes associated with inflammation, stress response, and cell proliferation.

2. Inflammatory Responses

Inflammation plays a significant role in IC/BPS, and several key mechanisms drive the inflammatory response within the bladder:

1. **Immune Cell Infiltration:**
   - **Mast Cells:** Mast cells are prominent in the bladder tissue of IC/BPS patients. They release histamine, proteases, and other mediators that contribute to inflammation and pain. Increased mast cell density in the bladder wall is a hallmark of IC/BPS.

- **Macrophages and T Cells:** The infiltration of macrophages and T cells into the bladder wall can perpetuate the inflammatory response, release cytokines, and contribute to tissue damage.

2. **Cytokine Release:**
   - **Pro-inflammatory Cytokines:** Elevated levels of pro-inflammatory cytokines such as tumor necrosis factor-alpha (TNF-α), interleukin-6 (IL-6), and interleukin-8 (IL-8) have been observed in IC/BPS. These cytokines promote inflammation and exacerbate pain and bladder dysfunction.
   - **Growth Factors:** Altered levels of growth factors, such as transforming growth factor-beta (TGF-β), can impact tissue repair and fibrosis, contributing to changes in bladder structure and function.

3. **Inflammatory Mediators:**
   - **Substance P:** Substance P, a neuropeptide associated with pain transmission, is often elevated in IC/BPS. It can interact with sensory nerves in the bladder wall, contributing to the sensation of pain and discomfort.
   - **Prostaglandins:** Prostaglandins, which are involved in the inflammatory response, may be increased in IC/BPS and contribute to bladder pain and discomfort.

3. Neurogenic Factors

The interaction between the bladder and the nervous system is a critical component of IC/BPS, with several neurogenic factors influencing symptom development:

1. **Neuroplasticity:**

    ◦ **Sensory Nerve Alterations:** In IC/BPS, sensory nerves in the bladder wall may undergo neuroplastic changes, leading to increased sensitivity and altered pain perception. These changes can result in heightened pain responses to normally non-painful stimuli.

    ◦ **Nerve Growth Factors:** Elevated levels of nerve growth factors, such as brain-derived neurotrophic factor (BDNF) and nerve growth factor (NGF), may contribute to the proliferation of sensory nerves and enhanced pain sensitivity.

2. **Pain Pathways:**

    ◦ **Central Sensitization:** IC/BPS is associated with central sensitization, a condition where the central nervous system becomes overly responsive to sensory input. This can result in the amplification of pain signals and contribute to chronic pain symptoms.

    ◦ **Cross-Talk Between Nerves and Immune Cells:** Interactions between sensory nerves and immune cells can exacerbate the inflammatory response and contribute to the sensation of pain.

4. Bladder Tissue Remodeling

Changes in bladder tissue structure and composition can significantly impact bladder function in IC/BPS:

1. **Fibrosis:**

    ◦ **Collagen Deposition:** Increased collagen deposition and fibrosis in the bladder wall can lead to decreased bladder compliance and increased stiffness. This remodeling alters the bladder's ability to stretch and can contribute to symptoms such as urgency and frequency.

- **Matrix Metalloproteinases (MMPs):** Elevated levels of MMPs, which are enzymes involved in extracellular matrix remodeling, can contribute to tissue degradation and fibrosis in IC/BPS.

2. **Cellular Proliferation and Apoptosis:**
   - **Cell Proliferation:** Increased proliferation of fibroblasts and other cells can contribute to bladder wall thickening and fibrosis. This proliferation may be driven by inflammatory cytokines and growth factors.

   - **Apoptosis:** Increased apoptosis of urothelial cells and other bladder cells can exacerbate the loss of barrier function and contribute to ongoing tissue damage.

5. Genetic and Epigenetic Factors

Genetic and epigenetic factors may influence susceptibility to IC/BPS and the severity of symptoms:

1. **Genetic Variants:**
   - **Susceptibility Genes:** Certain genetic variants may predispose individuals to IC/BPS by affecting bladder function, inflammatory responses, or pain perception. Research into susceptibility genes aims to identify potential biomarkers and therapeutic targets.

2. **Epigenetic Modifications:**
   - **DNA Methylation and Histone Modification:** Epigenetic changes, such as DNA methylation and histone modifications, can alter gene expression without changing the DNA sequence. These modifications may impact

inflammatory responses, cell growth, and tissue repair in IC/BPS.

6. Clinical Implications and Management

Understanding the cellular and molecular mechanisms underlying IC/BPS has important implications for diagnosis and treatment:

1. **Diagnostic Approaches:**
   - **Biomarkers:** Identifying biomarkers associated with urothelial dysfunction, inflammation, and neurogenic factors can aid in the diagnosis and monitoring of IC/BPS. Biomarkers may include cytokines, growth factors, and neuropeptides.

2. **Treatment Strategies:**
   - **Pharmacological Interventions:** Treatments targeting inflammation, pain, and urothelial barrier function are central to managing IC/BPS. These may include anti-inflammatory drugs, pain modulators, and agents that protect the bladder lining.

   - **Behavioral and Physical Therapies:** Behavioral therapies, such as bladder training and stress management, can complement pharmacological treatments. Physical therapies, including pelvic floor exercises, may help improve bladder function and alleviate symptoms.

Conclusion

The cellular and molecular mechanisms underlying Interstitial Cystitis/Bladder Pain Syndrome (IC/BPS) are complex and multifaceted, involving urothelial dysfunction, inflammatory responses, neurogenic factors, and changes in bladder tissue structure. A thorough understanding of these mechanisms is crucial for diagnosing and managing IC/BPS effectively. Advances in research continue to shed light on the intricate interplay of these factors, offering hope for the development of targeted therapies and improved patient outcomes.

Inflammatory Pathways and Mediators in Interstitial Cystitis/ Bladder Pain Syndrome (IC/BPS)

Interstitial Cystitis/Bladder Pain Syndrome (IC/BPS) is a chronic condition characterized by bladder pain, urgency, and frequency, with a significant inflammatory component contributing to its pathogenesis. Understanding the inflammatory pathways and mediators involved in IC/BPS is crucial for developing effective treatments and managing the symptoms associated with this debilitating condition. This section explores the key inflammatory pathways and mediators involved in IC/BPS, highlighting their roles in the disease process and their potential as therapeutic targets.

1. Inflammatory Pathways in IC/BPS

Inflammation in IC/BPS involves a complex interplay of cellular and molecular components that drive the chronic inflammatory response and contribute to bladder dysfunction. Key inflammatory pathways include:

1. **Toll-like Receptor (TLR) Pathway:**
   - **Activation:** Toll-like receptors are pattern recognition receptors located on the surface of immune cells and urothelial cells. They recognize pathogen-associated molecular patterns (PAMPs) and damage-associated molecular patterns (DAMPs), initiating an inflammatory response.
   - **Role in IC/BPS:** In IC/BPS, TLRs may be activated by urinary irritants or endogenous ligands, leading to the release of pro-

inflammatory cytokines and the recruitment of immune cells. This activation contributes to bladder inflammation and pain.

2. **Nuclear Factor-kappa B (NF-κB) Pathway:**
   - **Activation:** NF-κB is a transcription factor that regulates the expression of various inflammatory genes. It is activated in response to various stimuli, including cytokines, stress, and pathogens.
   - **Role in IC/BPS:** In IC/BPS, the NF-κB pathway is often activated, leading to increased expression of pro-inflammatory cytokines and adhesion molecules. This activation contributes to chronic inflammation, immune cell recruitment, and tissue damage.

3. **Inflammasome Pathway:**
   - **Activation:** The inflammasome is a multiprotein complex that activates inflammatory caspases, leading to the production of active interleukin-1β (IL-1β) and interleukin-18 (IL-18). This pathway plays a role in the innate immune response to cellular stress and damage.
   - **Role in IC/BPS:** In IC/BPS, activation of the inflammasome can lead to increased production of IL-1β, which contributes to inflammation and pain. This pathway is involved in the regulation of the inflammatory response and may be a target for therapeutic intervention.

4. **Mast Cell Activation:**
   - **Mechanism:** Mast cells are immune cells that contain granules with inflammatory mediators such as histamine, heparin, and

proteases. They play a key role in allergic reactions and inflammation.

- ◦ **Role in IC/BPS:** In IC/BPS, mast cells are often activated and infiltrate the bladder tissue. They release mediators that contribute to inflammation, pain, and bladder dysfunction. Mast cell activation is associated with increased bladder sensitivity and pain symptoms.

2. Inflammatory Mediators in IC/BPS

Several inflammatory mediators are involved in the pathogenesis of IC/BPS, playing crucial roles in driving the inflammatory response and contributing to the clinical manifestations of the disease. Key mediators include:

1. **Cytokines:**

   - ◦ **Tumor Necrosis Factor-alpha (TNF-α):** TNF-α is a pro-inflammatory cytokine produced by various cells, including macrophages and mast cells. It plays a central role in the inflammatory response by promoting the activation of other immune cells and the production of additional inflammatory mediators.

     - ▪ **Role in IC/BPS:** Elevated levels of TNF-α have been observed in the bladder tissue and urine of IC/BPS patients. TNF-α contributes to inflammation, pain, and tissue damage in IC/BPS.

   - ◦ **Interleukin-6 (IL-6):** IL-6 is a cytokine with both pro-inflammatory and anti-inflammatory properties. It is involved in the regulation of immune responses and the production of acute-phase proteins.

     - ▪ **Role in IC/BPS:** Increased levels of

IL-6 in IC/BPS are associated with inflammation and pain. IL-6 promotes the inflammatory response and may contribute to the chronic nature of the disease.

- **Interleukin-8 (IL-8):** IL-8 is a chemokine that attracts neutrophils to sites of inflammation. It is produced by various cells, including urothelial cells and immune cells.
  - **Role in IC/BPS:** Elevated levels of IL-8 in the bladder tissue and urine of IC/BPS patients indicate ongoing inflammation and immune cell recruitment. IL-8 contributes to the inflammatory environment and exacerbates bladder symptoms.

2. **Neuropeptides:**
   - **Substance P:** Substance P is a neuropeptide involved in pain transmission and inflammation. It is released from sensory nerves and immune cells in response to injury or irritation.
     - **Role in IC/BPS:** Increased levels of substance P are found in the bladder tissue of IC/BPS patients. It interacts with sensory neurons, contributing to pain and discomfort. Substance P is also involved in mast cell activation and inflammation.

3. **Prostaglandins:**
   - **Production:** Prostaglandins are lipid compounds derived from arachidonic acid and produced by cyclooxygenase enzymes (COX-1 and COX-2). They play a role in the inflammatory response and pain sensation.
     - **Role in IC/BPS:** Elevated levels

of prostaglandins, particularly prostaglandin E2 (PGE2), are associated with increased bladder pain and inflammation in IC/BPS. Prostaglandins sensitize sensory nerves and enhance the inflammatory response.

4. **Matrix Metalloproteinases (MMPs):**
    - **Function:** MMPs are enzymes responsible for the degradation of extracellular matrix components. They play a role in tissue remodeling and repair.
        - **Role in IC/BPS:** Increased expression of MMPs, such as MMP-2 and MMP-9, is observed in IC/BPS. These enzymes contribute to bladder tissue remodeling, fibrosis, and increased permeability, exacerbating bladder symptoms.

3. Interactions Between Inflammatory Pathways and Mediators

The interactions between various inflammatory pathways and mediators contribute to the chronic inflammation and symptoms observed in IC/BPS. Key interactions include:

1. **Crosstalk Between Cytokines and Neuropeptides:**
    - **Inflammatory Cytokines and Substance P:** Pro-inflammatory cytokines, such as TNF-α and IL-6, can enhance the release of substance P from sensory nerves and mast cells. This crosstalk amplifies the inflammatory response and contributes to pain and discomfort in IC/BPS.

2. **Mast Cell Activation and Cytokine Release:**
    - **Mast Cells and Cytokines:** Activated mast cells release cytokines and mediators that

further promote inflammation. The release of histamine and proteases from mast cells can increase the production of cytokines like TNF-α and IL-6, creating a feedback loop that perpetuates the inflammatory response.

3. **Prostaglandins and Cytokines:**
   - **Prostaglandins and Cytokine Production:** Prostaglandins, particularly PGE2, can enhance the production of pro-inflammatory cytokines, such as TNF-α and IL-6. This interaction contributes to the amplification of inflammation and pain in IC/BPS.

4. Therapeutic Implications

Understanding the inflammatory pathways and mediators involved in IC/BPS provides insights into potential therapeutic strategies:

1. **Targeting Inflammatory Pathways:**
   - **Pharmacological Inhibitors:** Drugs that target specific inflammatory pathways, such as TNF-α inhibitors or COX-2 inhibitors, may help reduce inflammation and alleviate symptoms in IC/BPS. These therapies aim to block the production or action of key inflammatory mediators.

2. **Mast Cell Stabilizers:**
   - **Treatment Options:** Mast cell stabilizers, such as cromolyn sodium, can help reduce mast cell activation and the release of inflammatory mediators. These agents may provide symptom relief by targeting one of the key sources of inflammation in IC/BPS.

3. **Neuropeptide Modulation:**
   - **Substance P Antagonists:** Drugs that block the action of substance P or its receptors may

help reduce pain and inflammation associated with IC/BPS. These therapies aim to interrupt the pain signaling pathways and alleviate symptoms.

4. **Biomarkers for Diagnosis and Monitoring:**
   ◦ **Inflammatory Mediators as Biomarkers:** Measuring levels of inflammatory mediators, such as cytokines, neuropeptides, and prostaglandins, may aid in the diagnosis and monitoring of IC/BPS. Biomarkers can provide information on disease activity and response to treatment.

Conclusion

Inflammatory pathways and mediators play a central role in the pathogenesis of Interstitial Cystitis/Bladder Pain Syndrome (IC/BPS). The complex interactions between cytokines, neuropeptides, and other inflammatory mediators contribute to the chronic inflammation and symptoms experienced by patients. Understanding these mechanisms provides valuable insights into potential therapeutic strategies and highlights the importance of targeted treatments to manage inflammation and improve patient outcomes. Ongoing research into the molecular and cellular aspects of IC/BPS will continue to enhance our knowledge and guide the development of more effective therapies for this challenging condition.

Pain Pathways and Neurotransmitters in Interstitial Cystitis/ Bladder Pain Syndrome (IC/BPS)

Pain is a hallmark symptom of Interstitial Cystitis/Bladder Pain Syndrome (IC/BPS), a chronic and often debilitating condition characterized by pelvic pain, urinary frequency, and urgency. The mechanisms underlying pain in IC/BPS involve complex interactions between pain pathways, neurotransmitters, and neuroplastic changes. Understanding these mechanisms is crucial for developing effective treatments and improving patient outcomes. This section explores the key pain pathways and neurotransmitters involved in IC/BPS, highlighting their roles in the development and maintenance of pain symptoms.

1. Pain Pathways in IC/BPS

Pain perception involves a series of pathways that transmit and modulate pain signals from the bladder to the brain. In IC/BPS, these pathways can be altered, leading to increased pain sensitivity and chronic discomfort. Key components of the pain pathways include:

1. **Peripheral Sensory Nerves:**
   - **Afferent Nerves:** Sensory nerve fibers in the bladder wall, including A-delta and C fibers, play a crucial role in detecting and transmitting pain signals. A-delta fibers are responsible for sharp, well-localized pain, while C fibers are associated with dull, diffuse pain.
   - **Bladder Sensory Receptors:** These receptors, including nociceptors and mechanoreceptors, are sensitive to mechanical stretch, chemical irritants, and inflammatory mediators. In IC/BPS, these receptors may become sensitized or dysfunctional, leading to increased pain perception.

2. **Spinal Cord Processing:**
   - **Dorsal Horn Neurons:** Pain signals from the bladder are transmitted to the spinal cord via the dorsal horn neurons. These neurons play a critical role in processing and modulating pain information before it is relayed to the brain.
   - **Central Sensitization:** In IC/BPS, central

sensitization can occur in the spinal cord, where neurons become hyperresponsive to sensory input. This heightened sensitivity contributes to the amplification of pain signals and the development of chronic pain.

3. **Supraspinal Processing:**
   - **Brain Structures:** Pain signals are further processed in various brain structures, including the thalamus, somatosensory cortex, and limbic system. These areas are involved in the perception, interpretation, and emotional aspects of pain.
   - **Pain Modulation:** The brain's ability to modulate pain signals through descending pathways can influence pain perception. Dysregulation of these pathways in IC/BPS may impair the brain's capacity to dampen or inhibit pain.

2. Neurotransmitters in IC/BPS

Neurotransmitters play a critical role in transmitting pain signals and modulating pain perception. In IC/BPS, alterations in neurotransmitter systems can contribute to the development and persistence of pain symptoms. Key neurotransmitters involved in IC/BPS include:

1. **Substance P:**
   - **Role:** Substance P is a neuropeptide involved in the transmission of pain signals. It is released from sensory nerves and contributes to the sensation of pain by interacting with neurokinin-1 (NK1) receptors.
   - **In IC/BPS:** Increased levels of substance P are found in the bladder tissue and urine of IC/BPS patients. Elevated substance P levels contribute to pain sensitivity, bladder

inflammation, and mast cell activation. Targeting substance P or its receptors may help alleviate pain symptoms.

2. **Calcitonin Gene-Related Peptide (CGRP):**
   ◦ **Role:** CGRP is another neuropeptide involved in pain transmission and inflammation. It is released from sensory neurons and acts as a potent vasodilator, contributing to neurogenic inflammation.
   ◦ **In IC/BPS:** Elevated CGRP levels have been observed in the bladder tissue of IC/BPS patients. CGRP contributes to bladder pain and increased blood flow to the bladder wall, exacerbating inflammation and discomfort.

3. **Glutamate:**
   ◦ **Role:** Glutamate is the primary excitatory neurotransmitter in the central nervous system. It plays a crucial role in the transmission of pain signals and the development of central sensitization.
   ◦ **In IC/BPS:** Dysregulation of glutamate signaling can contribute to central sensitization and chronic pain in IC/BPS. Elevated glutamate levels in the spinal cord and brain regions involved in pain processing may enhance pain perception and contribute to the persistence of symptoms.

4. **Serotonin:**
   ◦ **Role:** Serotonin is a neurotransmitter involved in the modulation of pain and mood. It acts on various receptors, including 5-HT3 and 5-HT7, to influence pain perception and emotional responses.
   ◦ **In IC/BPS:** Altered serotonin signaling may

contribute to pain sensitivity and affective symptoms in IC/BPS. Changes in serotonin levels or receptor function can impact the perception of pain and the emotional response to bladder discomfort.

5. **Endogenous Opioids:**
   ○ **Role:** Endogenous opioids, including endorphins and enkephalins, act as natural analgesics by binding to opioid receptors and modulating pain signals.

   ○ **In IC/BPS:** Dysregulation of the endogenous opioid system may contribute to pain in IC/BPS. Reduced opioid receptor function or altered opioid peptide levels can impair the body's ability to modulate pain and contribute to chronic discomfort.

3. Neuroplasticity and Central Sensitization

Neuroplasticity refers to the ability of the nervous system to adapt and reorganize in response to injury or chronic stimulation. In IC/BPS, neuroplastic changes contribute to central sensitization and the development of chronic pain.

1. **Central Sensitization:**
   ○ **Definition:** Central sensitization is a process in which the central nervous system becomes hyperresponsive to sensory input, leading to an amplification of pain signals.

   ○ **Mechanisms:** Changes in spinal cord and brain processing, including increased excitability of dorsal horn neurons and alterations in brain pain processing areas, contribute to central sensitization. Neuroplastic changes in response to chronic pain can lead to heightened pain sensitivity and persistent discomfort.

2. **Structural Changes:**
    - **Gray Matter Changes:** Structural imaging studies have shown alterations in gray matter density in brain regions involved in pain processing and emotional regulation in IC/BPS patients. These changes may reflect neuroplastic adaptations associated with chronic pain.
    - **Spinal Cord Changes:** Structural and functional changes in the spinal cord, including increased neuronal activity and alterations in pain processing circuits, contribute to central sensitization and chronic pain in IC/BPS.

4. Implications for Treatment

Understanding the pain pathways and neurotransmitters involved in IC/BPS has important implications for treatment strategies:

1. **Pharmacological Interventions:**
    - **Pain Modulators:** Medications targeting neurotransmitter systems, such as tricyclic antidepressants, selective serotonin reuptake inhibitors (SSRIs), and anticonvulsants, may help manage pain by modulating neurotransmitter levels and reducing central sensitization.
    - **Substance P Antagonists:** Drugs that block substance P or its receptors, such as NK1 receptor antagonists, may provide relief from bladder pain and inflammation in IC/BPS.

2. **Neuroplasticity-Based Therapies:**
    - **Neuromodulation:** Techniques such as transcranial magnetic stimulation (TMS) and spinal cord stimulation aim to modulate

pain processing pathways and reduce central sensitization. These therapies target neuroplastic changes associated with chronic pain.

○ **Cognitive-Behavioral Therapy (CBT):** CBT and other psychological interventions can help patients manage pain-related distress and improve coping strategies. Addressing the emotional and cognitive aspects of pain can enhance overall treatment outcomes.

3. **Lifestyle and Behavioral Approaches:**
   ○ **Bladder Training:** Bladder training and physical therapy may help improve bladder function and reduce pain by addressing the underlying mechanisms of bladder dysfunction and pain.

   ○ **Stress Management:** Stress reduction techniques, such as mindfulness and relaxation exercises, can help manage pain and improve quality of life by reducing the impact of stress on pain perception.

Conclusion

Pain pathways and neurotransmitters play a central role in the development and maintenance of pain in Interstitial Cystitis/ Bladder Pain Syndrome (IC/BPS). The complex interactions between peripheral and central pain processing systems, along with alterations in neurotransmitter signaling, contribute to the chronic pain experienced by patients. Understanding these mechanisms provides valuable insights into potential treatment strategies, including pharmacological interventions, neuroplasticity-based therapies, and lifestyle modifications. Advances in research and therapeutic approaches continue to enhance our ability to manage pain and improve the quality of life for individuals with IC/BPS.

Genetic and Epigenetic Factors in Interstitial Cystitis/Bladder Pain Syndrome (IC/BPS)

Interstitial Cystitis/Bladder Pain Syndrome (IC/BPS) is a complex and multifactorial condition characterized by chronic bladder pain, urinary urgency, and frequency, often without a clear infectious etiology. Recent research has highlighted the importance of genetic and epigenetic factors in the development and progression of IC/BPS. Understanding these factors can provide insights into the underlying mechanisms of the disease, identify potential biomarkers, and lead to the development of targeted therapies. This section explores the genetic and epigenetic factors involved in IC/BPS, focusing on their roles in disease susceptibility, progression, and therapeutic implications.

1. Genetic Factors

Genetic factors contribute to the susceptibility and severity of IC/BPS by influencing various biological processes, including bladder function, immune response, and pain perception. Key genetic aspects of IC/BPS include:

1. **Genetic Susceptibility:**
   - **Family History:** Evidence from familial and twin studies suggests a genetic predisposition to IC/BPS. Individuals with a family history of IC/BPS or related conditions may be at higher risk of developing the disease.
   - **Genetic Variants:** Genome-wide association studies (GWAS) have identified several genetic variants associated with IC/BPS. These variants are often located in genes involved in inflammation, tissue repair, and pain modulation.

2. **Specific Genes and Polymorphisms:**

◦ **TNF-α Gene:** The tumor necrosis factor-alpha (TNF-α) gene, which encodes a key pro-inflammatory cytokine, has been implicated in IC/BPS. Polymorphisms in the TNF-α gene may affect cytokine production and contribute to the inflammatory response observed in IC/BPS.

◦ **IL-6 Gene:** Interleukin-6 (IL-6) is another cytokine involved in inflammation and pain. Genetic variants in the IL-6 gene may influence cytokine levels and contribute to the development of IC/BPS.

◦ **GTPase Gene:** Variants in the GTPase gene, which is involved in cell signaling and immune response, have been associated with IC/BPS. These genetic variants may affect cellular responses to stress and inflammation.

3. **Gene-Environment Interactions:**

◦ **Environmental Triggers:** Genetic susceptibility to IC/BPS may be influenced by environmental factors such as infections, stress, and exposure to irritants. Interactions between genetic predispositions and environmental triggers can contribute to the development and exacerbation of IC/BPS.

2. Epigenetic Factors

Epigenetic modifications involve changes in gene expression without altering the DNA sequence itself. These modifications can affect cellular processes and contribute to disease development. Key epigenetic factors in IC/BPS include:

1. **DNA Methylation:**

◦ **Mechanism:** DNA methylation involves the addition of methyl groups to cytosine residues in the DNA, leading to changes in gene expression. Aberrant DNA methylation can affect genes involved in inflammation, pain perception, and bladder function.

- In IC/BPS: Changes in DNA methylation patterns have been observed in the bladder tissue of IC/BPS patients. These alterations may affect the expression of genes involved in the inflammatory response, tissue repair, and pain processing.

2. **Histone Modifications:**

- **Mechanism:** Histone modifications, such as acetylation and methylation, influence the accessibility of DNA and regulate gene expression. These modifications play a crucial role in chromatin remodeling and gene regulation.

- **In IC/BPS:** Alterations in histone modifications can impact the expression of genes associated with inflammation and pain. Changes in histone acetylation and methylation may contribute to the chronic inflammatory environment and pain symptoms in IC/BPS.

3. **Non-Coding RNAs:**

- **MicroRNAs (miRNAs):** miRNAs are small non-coding RNAs that regulate gene expression by binding to messenger RNAs (mRNAs) and promoting their degradation or inhibiting their translation. miRNAs play a role in various biological processes, including inflammation and pain.

  - **In IC/BPS:** Dysregulation of miRNAs has been observed in IC/BPS. Specific miRNAs may target genes involved in inflammation, pain signaling, and bladder function, contributing to the pathogenesis of the disease.

○ **Long Non-Coding RNAs (lncRNAs):** lncRNAs are long non-coding RNAs that regulate gene expression at the transcriptional and post-transcriptional levels. They play a role in cellular processes such as inflammation and stress response.

▪ **In IC/BPS:** Altered expression of lncRNAs in IC/BPS may impact the regulation of genes involved in inflammation and pain. lncRNAs may serve as potential biomarkers or therapeutic targets for IC/BPS.

3. Implications for Diagnosis and Treatment

Understanding genetic and epigenetic factors in IC/BPS has important implications for diagnosis, treatment, and personalized medicine:

1. **Genetic Biomarkers:**

○ **Identification:** Genetic biomarkers associated with IC/BPS may aid in the diagnosis and prognosis of the disease. Identifying genetic variants related to susceptibility and disease severity can provide insights into individual risk profiles and guide treatment decisions.

○ **Personalized Medicine:** Genetic information can be used to tailor treatments based on an individual's genetic makeup. Personalized approaches may improve treatment efficacy and reduce adverse effects by targeting specific genetic pathways involved in IC/BPS.

2. **Epigenetic Modifications as Therapeutic Targets:**

○ **Epigenetic Drugs:** Pharmacological agents that target epigenetic modifications, such as DNA methyltransferase inhibitors and histone deacetylase inhibitors, may offer potential therapeutic strategies for IC/BPS. These drugs can reverse abnormal epigenetic changes and restore normal gene expression.

- ○ **miRNA and lncRNA Therapies:** Therapeutic strategies targeting specific miRNAs or lncRNAs may modulate gene expression and inflammatory pathways involved in IC/BPS. RNA-based therapies, such as miRNA mimics or inhibitors, hold promise for the treatment of IC/BPS.

3. **Environmental and Lifestyle Modifications:**
   - ○ **Lifestyle Interventions:** Understanding gene-environment interactions can inform lifestyle and environmental modifications that may reduce disease risk and improve symptoms. Strategies such as stress management, dietary changes, and avoidance of irritants may complement pharmacological treatments.

4. Future Directions

Ongoing research into the genetic and epigenetic factors of IC/BPS holds promise for advancing our understanding of the disease and developing novel therapeutic approaches:

1. **Functional Genomics:**
   - ○ **Gene Function Studies:** Investigating the functional roles of specific genetic variants and epigenetic modifications in IC/BPS can provide insights into disease mechanisms and identify new therapeutic targets.

2. **Integration of Multi-Omics Data:**
   - ○ **Omics Approaches:** Integrating genomic, transcriptomic, epigenomic, and proteomic

data can offer a comprehensive understanding of IC/BPS and reveal interactions between genetic and epigenetic factors. Multi-omics approaches can facilitate the identification of biomarkers and therapeutic targets.

3. **Longitudinal Studies:**
    ◦ **Disease Progression:** Longitudinal studies examining genetic and epigenetic changes over time can provide insights into disease progression and treatment response. Understanding how genetic and epigenetic factors evolve with disease progression may inform personalized treatment strategies.

Conclusion

Genetic and epigenetic factors play a significant role in the development and progression of Interstitial Cystitis/ Bladder Pain Syndrome (IC/BPS). Genetic susceptibility, gene-environment interactions, and epigenetic modifications contribute to the pathogenesis of the disease by influencing inflammation, pain perception, and bladder function. Understanding these factors provides valuable insights into disease mechanisms, diagnostic approaches, and therapeutic strategies. Advances in genetic and epigenetic research continue to enhance our ability to diagnose, treat, and manage IC/ BPS, offering hope for improved outcomes and personalized medicine.

CHAPTER 3: CLINICAL PRESENTATION AND DIAGNOSIS

Symptoms and Their Variability in Interstitial Cystitis/ Bladder Pain Syndrome (IC/BPS)

Interstitial Cystitis/Bladder Pain Syndrome (IC/BPS) is a complex and multifaceted condition characterized by a range of symptoms affecting the bladder and its associated structures. The symptoms of IC/BPS can vary significantly between individuals, both in terms of presentation and severity. This variability poses challenges for diagnosis and treatment, and understanding the spectrum of symptoms is essential for effective management. This section explores the core symptoms of IC/BPS, their variability, and the factors contributing to this variability.

1. Core Symptoms of IC/BPS

IC/BPS is defined by several key symptoms, which may overlap with those of other urological and gynecological conditions. The core symptoms include:

1. **Bladder Pain:**
   - **Description:** Persistent pain or discomfort in the bladder area is a hallmark symptom of IC/BPS. The pain may be localized to the suprapubic region but can also radiate to the lower abdomen, pelvis, or lower back.

- ◦ **Characteristics:** The pain may be described as aching, burning, or sharp and can vary in intensity. It is often exacerbated by bladder filling and relieved by urination, although some patients experience pain even after voiding.

2. **Urinary Frequency:**
   - ◦ **Description:** Increased urinary frequency is a common symptom in IC/BPS. Patients may feel the need to urinate more frequently than usual, with some individuals reporting voiding every hour or more frequently.
   - ◦ **Characteristics:** Urinary frequency can be accompanied by urgency and may interfere with daily activities and quality of life. The increased frequency is often driven by bladder discomfort and the need to relieve pressure.

3. **Urgency:**
   - ◦ **Description:** Urinary urgency is characterized by a sudden and strong urge to urinate, which can be difficult to control. This symptom is often associated with the need to void immediately.
   - ◦ **Characteristics:** Urgency can be distressing and may lead to anxiety or avoidance behaviors. It is frequently reported alongside increased urinary frequency and can impact social and occupational functioning.

4. **Pain During or After Urination:**
   - ◦ **Description:** Some patients with IC/BPS experience pain or discomfort during or after urination. This symptom can be related to bladder inflammation or irritation.
   - ◦ **Characteristics:** Pain during or after

urination may be sharp or burning and can vary in intensity. It can be a significant source of distress for patients and may influence their hydration habits.

5. **Pelvic Pain:**
   - **Description:** In addition to bladder pain, many patients with IC/BPS report pelvic pain. This pain may extend beyond the bladder area to the pelvic floor muscles, vulva, or rectum.

   - **Characteristics:** Pelvic pain can be chronic and may be exacerbated by activities that involve pelvic pressure or muscle tension. It can be associated with conditions such as pelvic floor dysfunction or endometriosis.

2. Variability in Symptoms

The symptoms of IC/BPS can vary widely among individuals, both in terms of presentation and severity. Several factors contribute to this variability:

1. **Symptom Onset and Progression:**
   - **Onset:** The onset of IC/BPS symptoms can vary. For some individuals, symptoms may develop gradually over months or years, while others may experience a more abrupt onset.

   - **Progression:** The progression of symptoms can also differ. Some patients may experience a steady worsening of symptoms, while others may have fluctuating symptoms with periods of exacerbation and remission.

2. **Symptom Severity:**
   - **Mild to Severe:** IC/BPS symptoms can range from mild discomfort to severe pain. The severity of symptoms can influence an individual's daily functioning and quality of

life.

- ◦ **Variability:** Severity can fluctuate over time, with some patients experiencing significant symptom relief during certain periods and others facing persistent or worsening symptoms.

3. **Impact of Bladder Filling:**
   - ◦ **Symptom Triggering:** Bladder filling often triggers symptoms in IC/BPS. However, the degree to which bladder filling affects symptoms can vary among individuals.
   - ◦ **Relief After Urination:** While many patients find relief from symptoms after urination, some individuals may continue to experience pain or discomfort despite emptying the bladder.

4. **Associated Conditions:**
   - ◦ **Comorbidities:** IC/BPS is frequently associated with other conditions such as irritable bowel syndrome (IBS), fibromyalgia, and chronic pelvic pain syndrome. The presence of these comorbidities can influence the symptom profile and overall disease experience.
   - ◦ **Overlap with Other Conditions:** Symptoms of IC/BPS may overlap with those of other urological or gynecological conditions, making diagnosis and management more complex.

5. **Psychological and Emotional Factors:**
   - ◦ **Stress and Anxiety:** Psychological factors such as stress, anxiety, and depression can impact the perception and severity of IC/BPS symptoms. Emotional distress may

exacerbate pain and influence symptom reporting.

- ◦ **Coping Mechanisms:** Individual coping mechanisms and psychological resilience can also affect how symptoms are experienced and managed.

3. Factors Contributing to Symptom Variability

Several factors contribute to the variability in IC/BPS symptoms:

1. **Biological Factors:**
   - ◦ **Genetic Predisposition:** Genetic factors may influence the susceptibility to IC/BPS and the severity of symptoms. Variations in genes related to inflammation, pain perception, and bladder function can contribute to symptom variability.

   - ◦ **Hormonal Influences:** Hormonal fluctuations, particularly in women, can impact IC/BPS symptoms. Menstrual cycles, pregnancy, and menopause may influence symptom severity and progression.

2. **Inflammatory and Immunological Factors:**
   - ◦ **Inflammatory Response:** Variations in the inflammatory response can contribute to differences in symptom presentation and severity. Some individuals may have a more pronounced inflammatory response, leading to increased pain and discomfort.

   - ◦ **Immune System Function:** The role of the immune system in IC/BPS is complex and may vary among individuals. Differences in immune system function and regulation can affect symptom experience.

3. **Bladder Pathology:**

- **Bladder Wall Changes:** Structural changes in the bladder wall, such as epithelial damage or fibrosis, can influence symptom presentation. The extent and location of these changes may contribute to variability in pain and urinary symptoms.

- **Bladder Capacity:** Variations in bladder capacity and compliance can affect symptom severity. Some patients may have a reduced bladder capacity, leading to more frequent and urgent urination.

4. **Lifestyle and Environmental Factors:**
   - **Diet and Fluid Intake:** Dietary factors and fluid intake can impact IC/BPS symptoms. Certain foods and beverages may exacerbate symptoms, while hydration practices may influence bladder function.

   - **Activity Level:** Physical activity and lifestyle choices can affect symptom severity. Activities that involve pelvic pressure or strain may exacerbate symptoms, while regular exercise may improve overall well-being.

4. Management and Treatment Considerations

The variability in IC/BPS symptoms necessitates a personalized approach to management and treatment. Key considerations include:

1. **Individualized Treatment Plans:**
   - **Symptom Targeting:** Treatment plans should be tailored to address the specific symptoms and severity experienced by each patient. This may involve a combination of pharmacological and non-pharmacological therapies.

- **Multidisciplinary Approach:** A multidisciplinary approach involving urologists, pain specialists, physical therapists, and mental health professionals can help address the diverse aspects of IC/BPS.

2. **Monitoring and Adjustment:**
   - **Symptom Tracking:** Regular monitoring of symptoms and treatment response is essential. Patients should be encouraged to track their symptoms, including pain levels, urinary frequency, and triggers.

   - **Treatment Adjustments:** Treatment plans may need to be adjusted based on changes in symptom severity or new developments. Flexibility in treatment approaches can help manage variability effectively.

3. **Patient Education and Support:**
   - **Education:** Providing education about IC/BPS and its management can empower patients to make informed decisions and actively participate in their care.

   - **Support:** Emotional and psychological support can help patients cope with the impact of IC/BPS on their daily lives. Support groups and counseling can provide valuable resources and coping strategies.

Conclusion

The symptoms of Interstitial Cystitis/Bladder Pain Syndrome (IC/BPS) are diverse and can vary widely among individuals. Core symptoms such as bladder pain, urinary frequency, urgency, pain during or after urination, and pelvic pain can differ in terms of onset, severity, and impact on daily functioning. The variability in symptoms is influenced by a range of factors, including biological, inflammatory, hormonal, and lifestyle factors. Understanding this variability is crucial for developing personalized treatment plans and improving patient outcomes. A comprehensive and individualized approach to management, along with ongoing monitoring and support, can help address the complex and variable nature of IC/BPS symptoms.

Diagnostic Criteria and Classification of Interstitial Cystitis/Bladder Pain Syndrome (IC/BPS)

Interstitial Cystitis/Bladder Pain Syndrome (IC/BPS) is a chronic condition characterized by bladder pain, urgency, and frequency. The diagnosis of IC/BPS is challenging due to the variability of symptoms and the overlap with other urological and gynecological conditions. Accurate diagnosis requires a thorough evaluation and a clear understanding of diagnostic criteria and classification systems. This section provides an in-depth overview of the diagnostic criteria and classification of IC/BPS, including the approaches used to distinguish it from other conditions and the current standards for diagnosis.

1. Diagnostic Criteria

The diagnosis of IC/BPS is primarily clinical, based on symptom presentation and the exclusion of other potential causes of bladder pain. Key diagnostic criteria include:

1. **Symptom-Based Criteria:**
   - **Bladder Pain:** Persistent or recurrent pain or discomfort in the bladder area, which can be described as aching, burning, or sharp. The pain may be localized to the suprapubic region and can radiate to the lower abdomen, pelvis, or lower back.

   - **Urinary Frequency and Urgency:** Increased urinary frequency (e.g., more than 8 times per day) and urgency to urinate. These symptoms must be associated with the pain or discomfort experienced by the patient.

- **Symptom Duration:** Symptoms should be present for at least 6 weeks to meet diagnostic criteria. Shorter durations may not be sufficient for a definitive diagnosis of IC/BPS.

2. **Exclusion of Other Conditions:**
   - **Rule Out Infection:** Diagnosis requires the exclusion of urinary tract infections (UTIs) and other infectious causes of bladder pain. Negative urine cultures and the absence of bacterial infection are essential for ruling out infection.

   - **Exclude Other Urological Conditions:** Conditions such as bladder cancer, bladder stones, and benign prostatic hyperplasia (BPH) should be ruled out through appropriate diagnostic tests. Cystoscopy and imaging studies may be used for this purpose.

   - **Evaluate for Gynecological Conditions:** In women, gynecological conditions such as endometriosis or pelvic inflammatory disease (PID) should be considered and excluded, as they can present with similar symptoms.

3. **Additional Diagnostic Tests:**
   - **Cystoscopy:** Cystoscopy allows for direct visualization of the bladder mucosa and can help identify characteristic findings such as Hunner's lesions or bladder mucosal abnormalities. However, the absence of these findings does not rule out IC/BPS.

   - **Urodynamic Studies:** Urodynamic testing can assess bladder function, capacity, and compliance. Abnormal findings may support the diagnosis of IC/BPS but are not definitive.

- **Biopsy:** In some cases, a bladder biopsy may be performed to evaluate for histological changes and rule out other conditions. Biopsy findings can provide additional diagnostic information.

2. Classification of IC/BPS

The classification of IC/BPS helps to differentiate between subtypes of the condition and guide treatment strategies. Two primary classification systems are commonly used:

1. **NIDDK Classification:**
   - **Description:** The National Institute of Diabetes and Digestive and Kidney Diseases (NIDDK) classification system is one of the most widely used for IC/BPS. It categorizes IC/BPS into two main subtypes based on cystoscopic findings and symptom patterns.

   - **Subtypes:**
     - **Type 1 (Interstitial Cystitis):** Characterized by the presence of Hunner's lesions, which are ulcers or inflamed patches on the bladder mucosa. This subtype may be associated with more severe symptoms and often requires different treatment approaches.

     - **Type 2 (Bladder Pain Syndrome without Hunner's Lesions):** Characterized by the absence of Hunner's lesions. This subtype includes patients with bladder pain and symptoms of frequency and urgency but without specific cystoscopic findings.

2. **IC/BPS Classification System:**
   - **Description:** The IC/BPS classification system divides the condition into distinct categories based on symptom severity, functional impact, and associated features.

   - **Categories:**
     - **Mild:** Symptoms are present but have minimal impact on daily life and functioning. Patients may experience occasional discomfort and increased urinary frequency without significant interference with daily activities.

     - **Moderate:** Symptoms have a moderate impact on daily life, with frequent pain, urgency, and urinary frequency. Patients may experience disruptions in work, social activities, and sleep.

     - **Severe:** Symptoms have a significant impact on quality of life, with persistent pain, frequent and urgent need to urinate, and severe disruption to daily activities. Patients may experience debilitating pain and a significant decrease in overall functioning.

3. Challenges in Diagnosis and Classification

The diagnosis and classification of IC/BPS present several challenges:

1. **Overlap with Other Conditions:**
   - **Symptom Similarities:** IC/BPS symptoms can overlap with those of other urological, gynecological, and gastrointestinal conditions, making differential diagnosis challenging. Conditions such as chronic pelvic

pain syndrome, irritable bowel syndrome (IBS), and endometriosis can present with similar symptoms.

- **Variability in Presentation:** The wide variability in symptoms and their severity can complicate diagnosis and classification. Patients may present with different combinations of symptoms, making it difficult to fit them into a specific category.

2. **Lack of Definitive Diagnostic Tests:**
   - **Absence of Biomarkers:** There are no definitive biomarkers for IC/BPS, and diagnosis relies on clinical assessment and exclusion of other conditions. The absence of specific biomarkers means that diagnosis is primarily based on symptom presentation and clinical judgment.
   - **Variability in Cystoscopic Findings:** Not all patients with IC/BPS exhibit characteristic cystoscopic findings such as Hunner's lesions. This variability can lead to challenges in classification and treatment planning.

3. **Need for Comprehensive Evaluation:**
   - **Multidisciplinary Approach:** Given the complexity of IC/BPS, a comprehensive evaluation by a multidisciplinary team may be necessary. Urologists, gynecologists, pain specialists, and other healthcare providers may collaborate to ensure an accurate diagnosis and effective management plan.

4. Management and Treatment Implications

The classification and accurate diagnosis of IC/BPS have important implications for management and treatment:

1. **Tailored Treatment Plans:**
   - **Subtype-Specific Approaches:** Treatment strategies may vary based on the subtype of IC/BPS. For example, patients with Hunner's lesions may benefit from specific interventions such as bladder instillations or cauterization, while those without Hunner's lesions may require different treatment approaches.

   - **Symptom-Based Management:** Management should be tailored to the specific symptoms and severity experienced by each patient. A combination of pharmacological, behavioral, and physical therapies may be employed to address the diverse aspects of IC/BPS.

2. **Monitoring and Follow-Up:**
   - **Regular Assessment:** Ongoing monitoring of symptoms and treatment response is essential. Patients should be regularly assessed to evaluate the effectiveness of treatment and make necessary adjustments.

   - **Patient Education:** Providing education about IC/BPS and its management can empower patients to actively participate in their care and make informed decisions about treatment options.

3. **Research and Advancements:**
   - **Ongoing Research:** Continued research into the pathophysiology of IC/BPS, as well as the development of new diagnostic and treatment approaches, is crucial for improving patient outcomes. Advances in research may lead to the identification of novel biomarkers and targeted therapies.

Conclusion

The diagnostic criteria and classification of Interstitial Cystitis/ Bladder Pain Syndrome (IC/BPS) are critical for accurate diagnosis and effective management. The core symptoms of bladder pain, urinary frequency, and urgency must be assessed in the context of excluding other conditions. Classification systems such as the NIDDK and IC/BPS classification help differentiate between subtypes and guide treatment strategies. Challenges in diagnosis include symptom overlap with other conditions and the lack of definitive biomarkers. A comprehensive and individualized approach to diagnosis and management is essential for addressing the complex nature of IC/BPS and improving patient outcomes.

Differential Diagnosis of Interstitial Cystitis/Bladder Pain Syndrome (IC/BPS)

The differential diagnosis of Interstitial Cystitis/Bladder Pain Syndrome (IC/BPS) is crucial due to the overlap of its symptoms with other urological, gynecological, and gastrointestinal conditions. Accurate diagnosis is essential for effective management and treatment. This section outlines the key conditions that must be considered when diagnosing IC/ BPS, along with their distinguishing features and diagnostic approaches.

1. Urological Conditions

1. **Urinary Tract Infection (UTI):**
   - **Symptoms:** UTIs can present with symptoms such as dysuria (painful urination), urinary frequency, urgency, and suprapubic pain.
   - **Diagnostic Approach:** Diagnosis is based on urine culture and sensitivity testing. A positive culture confirms bacterial infection, whereas a negative culture suggests other

causes for the symptoms.

2. **Bladder Cancer:**
   ◦ **Symptoms:** Bladder cancer may present with hematuria (blood in urine), dysuria, urinary frequency, and pelvic pain.
   ◦ **Diagnostic Approach:** Cystoscopy is used for direct visualization of the bladder and to obtain biopsy samples. Imaging studies such as ultrasound or CT scan can also aid in diagnosis.

3. **Bladder Stones:**
   ◦ **Symptoms:** Bladder stones can cause pain, urinary frequency, urgency, and hematuria.
   ◦ **Diagnostic Approach:** Diagnosis is typically confirmed with imaging studies such as ultrasound or X-ray. Cystoscopy can also identify and allow for the removal of bladder stones.

4. **Benign Prostatic Hyperplasia (BPH) (in males):**
   ◦ **Symptoms:** BPH can cause urinary frequency, urgency, and difficulty starting or stopping urination.
   ◦ **Diagnostic Approach:** Diagnosis is based on a combination of patient history, physical examination, including a digital rectal exam (DRE), and imaging studies such as transabdominal ultrasound.

5. **Urethral Syndrome:**
   ◦ **Symptoms:** This condition presents with symptoms similar to those of a UTI, including dysuria and urinary frequency, but without evidence of infection.
   ◦ **Diagnostic Approach:** Diagnosis is based on

symptom presentation and the exclusion of infection through negative urine cultures. Further evaluation may involve urethroscopy.

2. Gynecological Conditions

1. Endometriosis:

- **Symptoms:** Endometriosis can cause pelvic pain, dysmenorrhea (painful menstruation), dyspareunia (painful intercourse), and urinary symptoms.

- **Diagnostic Approach:** Diagnosis is typically made through pelvic ultrasound, MRI, or laparoscopy. Endometriosis is confirmed by direct visualization and biopsy during laparoscopy.

2. Pelvic Inflammatory Disease (PID):

- **Symptoms:** PID presents with pelvic pain, abnormal vaginal discharge, fever, and pain during intercourse.

- **Diagnostic Approach:** Diagnosis is based on clinical symptoms, pelvic examination, and laboratory tests. Imaging studies like pelvic ultrasound or laparoscopy may be used for further evaluation.

3. Vulvodynia:

- **Symptoms:** Vulvodynia is characterized by chronic pain or discomfort in the vulvar region, which may be associated with burning or itching.

- **Diagnostic Approach:** Diagnosis is made through patient history and physical examination. The presence of pain in the vulvar area, without an obvious cause, helps in distinguishing vulvodynia from other conditions.

3. Gastrointestinal Conditions

1. **Irritable Bowel Syndrome (IBS):**
   - **Symptoms:** IBS can present with abdominal pain, bloating, and changes in bowel habits, such as diarrhea or constipation.
   - **Diagnostic Approach:** Diagnosis is based on symptom patterns and the exclusion of other gastrointestinal disorders. Rome IV criteria are commonly used to diagnose IBS.

2. **Diverticulitis:**
   - **Symptoms:** Diverticulitis presents with lower abdominal pain, fever, and changes in bowel habits, such as constipation or diarrhea.
   - **Diagnostic Approach:** Diagnosis is typically confirmed with imaging studies such as a CT scan of the abdomen and pelvis, which can reveal diverticula and inflammation.

3. **Chronic Pelvic Pain Syndrome (CPPS):**
   - **Symptoms:** CPPS is characterized by chronic pelvic pain without an obvious cause, overlapping with symptoms of IC/BPS.
   - **Diagnostic Approach:** Diagnosis involves a comprehensive assessment to rule out other conditions. Evaluation may include a detailed history, physical examination, and diagnostic tests to exclude other potential causes.

4. Other Conditions

1. **Fibromyalgia:**
   - **Symptoms:** Fibromyalgia is associated with widespread musculoskeletal pain, fatigue, sleep disturbances, and sometimes bladder symptoms.

- **Diagnostic Approach:** Diagnosis is based on the presence of widespread pain and tender points. Exclusion of other conditions and a comprehensive evaluation of symptoms are essential.

2. **Chronic Prostatitis/Chronic Pelvic Pain Syndrome (CP/CPPS) (in males):**
    - **Symptoms:** CP/CPPS presents with pelvic pain, urinary symptoms, and sexual dysfunction. It can overlap with symptoms of IC/BPS.

    - **Diagnostic Approach:** Diagnosis involves a detailed history, physical examination, and sometimes prostate-specific antigen (PSA) testing. The absence of infection in prostate secretions helps differentiate it from bacterial prostatitis.

3. **Chronic Fatigue Syndrome (CFS):**
    - **Symptoms:** CFS is characterized by persistent fatigue that is not alleviated by rest and may be accompanied by pain, including pelvic pain.

    - **Diagnostic Approach:** Diagnosis is based on clinical criteria, including the presence of fatigue, post-exertional malaise, and other symptoms, following the exclusion of other conditions.

5. Diagnostic Approach and Management

Given the overlap of symptoms among various conditions, a thorough and systematic diagnostic approach is crucial:

1. **Detailed Patient History:**
    - **Symptom Onset and Duration:** Assess the onset, duration, and progression of

symptoms.

- **Associated Symptoms:** Identify any associated symptoms, such as gastrointestinal or gynecological symptoms, to aid in differential diagnosis.

2. **Physical Examination:**
   - **Pelvic Examination:** For female patients, a pelvic examination can help identify gynecological issues. For males, a digital rectal exam (DRE) is essential for assessing prostate health.
   - **Abdominal Examination:** An abdominal examination can identify signs of other conditions, such as diverticulitis.

3. **Laboratory and Imaging Studies:**
   - **Urinalysis and Urine Culture:** To rule out UTIs and other urinary tract conditions.
   - **Imaging Studies:** Ultrasound, CT scans, or MRI can help visualize structural abnormalities and guide diagnosis.
   - **Endoscopic Procedures:** Cystoscopy, laparoscopy, or colonoscopy may be used to directly visualize and assess specific areas.

4. **Multidisciplinary Evaluation:**
   - **Collaborative Care:** In complex cases, collaboration among urologists, gynecologists, gastroenterologists, and other specialists may be necessary to ensure comprehensive evaluation and management.

Conclusion

The differential diagnosis of Interstitial Cystitis/Bladder Pain Syndrome (IC/BPS) involves distinguishing it from a range of urological, gynecological, and gastrointestinal conditions that share similar symptoms. Accurate diagnosis requires a thorough evaluation, including detailed patient history, physical examination, and appropriate diagnostic tests. By considering and excluding other potential causes, clinicians can more effectively diagnose IC/BPS and develop tailored treatment plans to address the unique needs of each patient.

Diagnostic Tests and Procedures in Interstitial Cystitis/ Bladder Pain Syndrome (IC/BPS)

The diagnosis of Interstitial Cystitis/Bladder Pain Syndrome (IC/BPS) involves a comprehensive evaluation that includes various diagnostic tests and procedures. These tests help differentiate IC/BPS from other conditions with similar symptoms and assess the severity and extent of bladder involvement. This section delves into the primary diagnostic tests and procedures used in the evaluation of IC/BPS, including urinalysis and urine culture, cystoscopy and biopsy, urodynamics, and the potassium sensitivity test.

Urinalysis and Urine Culture

Urinalysis

Urinalysis is a fundamental diagnostic test used to assess the health of the urinary system and detect abnormalities. In the context of IC/BPS, urinalysis helps rule out other conditions such as urinary tract infections (UTIs) and kidney disorders.

- **Components of Urinalysis:**
    - **Physical Examination:** Observes the color, clarity, and odor of the urine. Normal urine is usually light yellow and clear. Changes in color or turbidity can indicate infection or other conditions.
    - **Chemical Analysis:** Uses dipstick tests to measure various substances in the urine, including:

- **pH:** Normal urine pH ranges from 4.5 to 8.0. An abnormal pH may indicate metabolic or systemic issues.

- **Protein:** The presence of protein (proteinuria) can suggest kidney damage or disease.

- **Glucose:** The presence of glucose (glycosuria) may indicate diabetes.

- **Blood:** Hematuria, or the presence of blood, can signal infection, stones, or trauma.

- **Nitrites and Leukocyte Esterase:** These markers can indicate bacterial infection. Positive nitrites and leukocyte esterase suggest a UTI, while negative results help rule out infection.

- **Interpretation:** In IC/BPS patients, urinalysis typically shows normal findings if there is no concurrent infection. An abnormal urinalysis prompts further diagnostic investigations to explore other potential causes of symptoms.

Urine Culture

Urine culture is a specific test used to identify bacterial infections and determine the appropriate antibiotic treatment. This test is crucial for distinguishing IC/BPS from conditions caused by bacterial pathogens.

- **Procedure:**
  - **Sample Collection:** A clean-catch midstream urine sample is collected to minimize contamination. In some cases, a catheterized sample may be required for more accurate results.
  - **Culturing:** The urine sample is inoculated

onto specialized culture media to promote bacterial growth. Incubation typically occurs at 35-37°C for 24-48 hours.

- **Results Interpretation:**
  - **Positive Culture:** Indicates the presence of pathogenic bacteria. The culture report identifies the bacterial species and their antibiotic susceptibility, guiding treatment.
  - **Negative Culture:** Suggests that bacteria are not responsible for the symptoms. A negative culture is a key factor in diagnosing IC/BPS, as it rules out bacterial infection.
- **Significance in IC/BPS:** A negative urine culture supports the diagnosis of IC/BPS by excluding infection as a cause of symptoms. Recurrent negative cultures in symptomatic patients can further reinforce the diagnosis.

Cystoscopy and Biopsy

Cystoscopy

Cystoscopy is a procedure that allows direct visualization of the bladder and urethra using a flexible or rigid cystoscope. It is instrumental in diagnosing IC/BPS and differentiating it from other urological conditions.

- **Procedure:**
  - **Preparation:** The patient may receive local or general anesthesia. A local anesthetic gel is often applied to the urethra to minimize discomfort.
  - **Insertion:** The cystoscope is gently inserted through the urethra and advanced into the bladder. The bladder is typically filled with sterile fluid to enhance visualization.
  - **Examination:** The urologist examines the bladder mucosa for abnormalities such

as inflammation, ulcers, or lesions. The procedure allows for direct assessment of bladder wall condition.

- **Findings in IC/BPS:**
  - **Hunner's Lesions:** Characteristic of Type 1 IC/BPS, Hunner's lesions appear as inflamed or ulcerated areas on the bladder mucosa. These lesions are indicative of more severe forms of IC/BPS.
  - **Other Abnormalities:** In patients with Type 2 IC/BPS (non-Hunner's), cystoscopy may reveal a normal bladder appearance or non-specific changes such as hyperemia (increased blood flow) and mucosal fissures.

Biopsy

During cystoscopy, a biopsy may be performed to obtain tissue samples for histological examination. This is particularly useful for ruling out malignancies and assessing bladder tissue changes.

- **Procedure:**
  - **Tissue Sampling:** Small samples of bladder tissue are collected using biopsy forceps or a brush. The procedure is usually done under local or general anesthesia.
  - **Histological Analysis:** The tissue samples are examined microscopically for signs of inflammation, fibrosis, or malignancy.

- **Significance:**
  - **Diagnosis of IC/BPS:** Histological findings in IC/BPS may show chronic inflammation and changes consistent with the condition. Biopsy results help rule out other potential causes, such as bladder cancer.
  - **Treatment Planning:** The presence of Hunner's lesions or significant inflammation

may influence treatment decisions, including the use of specific therapies such as bladder instillations or cauterization.

Urodynamics

Urodynamics

Urodynamic testing assesses bladder function, capacity, and compliance. These tests are crucial for understanding the functional aspects of the bladder and differentiating IC/BPS from other conditions affecting bladder function.

- **Types of Urodynamic Tests:**
  - **Uroflowmetry:** Measures the rate and volume of urine flow during voiding. It helps assess bladder emptying efficiency and can detect obstruction or bladder outlet dysfunction.
  - **Cystometry:** Evaluates bladder capacity, compliance, and detrusor pressure during filling and voiding. This test involves filling the bladder with a sterile fluid while measuring bladder pressure and sensation.
  - **Pressure-Flow Study:** Combines uroflowmetry and cystometry to assess the relationship between bladder pressure and urine flow. It helps diagnose detrusor-sphincter dyssynergia and other functional abnormalities.
  - **Electromyography (EMG):** Measures electrical activity in the pelvic floor muscles and sphincters. It can identify issues such as muscle dysfunction or abnormal sphincter activity.
- **Procedure:**
  - **Preparation:** The patient is asked to arrive with a full bladder. Local anesthetic gel may be applied to the urethra.

- **Testing:** A catheter is inserted into the bladder to fill it with fluid. Sensors measure bladder pressure, flow rate, and sensation.

- **Interpretation:**
  - **Normal Findings:** In IC/BPS, urodynamic studies often show normal bladder function, although some patients may have reduced bladder capacity or compliance.
  - **Abnormal Findings:** Urodynamic abnormalities may indicate other conditions, such as bladder outlet obstruction or detrusor overactivity. These findings help differentiate IC/BPS from other bladder disorders.

- **Significance in IC/BPS:**
  - **Functional Assessment:** Urodynamics provides insights into bladder function and helps identify any additional functional issues that may complicate IC/BPS.
  - **Treatment Planning:** Abnormal urodynamic findings can guide treatment decisions, such as the need for bladder training or other interventions.

Potassium Sensitivity Test

Potassium Sensitivity Test

The potassium sensitivity test is a diagnostic procedure used to assess bladder sensitivity to potassium, which is believed to be related to the inflammatory process in IC/BPS. This test helps identify individuals with a heightened sensitivity to potassium, a marker that may be associated with the condition.

- **Procedure:**
  - **Preparation:** The patient undergoes a standard cystoscopy procedure to allow for bladder instillation.
  - **Instillation:** A solution containing potassium

chloride is instilled into the bladder through a catheter. The test typically involves a 0.4% potassium chloride solution.

- ◦ **Assessment:** The patient is monitored for pain or discomfort during and after the instillation. The response is evaluated based on the onset and severity of symptoms.

- · **Interpretation:**
    - ◦ **Positive Test:** A positive response is indicated by a significant increase in pain or discomfort following the instillation of potassium chloride. This suggests heightened bladder sensitivity and may support a diagnosis of IC/BPS.

    - ◦ **Negative Test:** A negative response, where there is no significant increase in pain or discomfort, does not rule out IC/BPS but suggests that potassium sensitivity is not a primary factor in the patient's symptoms.

- · **Significance in IC/BPS:**
    - ◦ **Diagnostic Utility:** The potassium sensitivity test helps identify patients with increased bladder sensitivity, a feature that may be associated with IC/BPS. However, it is not a standalone diagnostic tool and should be used in conjunction with other diagnostic tests and clinical evaluation.

    - ◦ **Limitations:** The test is not universally available and may not be applicable to all patients. It is typically used as part of a broader diagnostic approach.

Conclusion

The diagnostic evaluation of Interstitial Cystitis/Bladder Pain Syndrome (IC/BPS) involves a combination of tests and procedures designed to rule out other conditions, assess bladder function, and identify characteristic features of the disease. Urinalysis and urine culture are foundational tests used to exclude infections, while cystoscopy and biopsy provide direct visualization and tissue analysis of the bladder. Urodynamic testing evaluates bladder function and capacity, helping to identify any functional abnormalities. The potassium sensitivity test assesses bladder sensitivity to potassium, which may be associated with IC/BPS.

Assessment Scales and Questionnaires for Interstitial Cystitis/Bladder Pain Syndrome (IC/BPS)

Assessment scales and questionnaires are pivotal tools in the evaluation and management of Interstitial Cystitis/Bladder Pain Syndrome (IC/BPS). They offer a structured approach to quantifying symptoms, assessing the impact on quality of life, and monitoring treatment efficacy. This section provides an in-depth exploration of various assessment scales and questionnaires used in the diagnosis and management of IC/BPS, including their purpose, administration, and relevance.

1. Purpose of Assessment Scales and Questionnaires

Assessment scales and questionnaires serve multiple functions in the context of IC/BPS:

- **Symptom Quantification:** They help quantify the severity of symptoms such as pain, urgency, and frequency, providing a baseline for comparison over time.
- **Quality of Life Evaluation:** They assess the impact of IC/BPS on daily life and overall well-being, including physical, emotional, and social aspects.
- **Treatment Monitoring:** They allow for the evaluation of treatment outcomes and the effectiveness of various therapeutic interventions.

- **Diagnostic Assistance:** They support the diagnostic process by capturing a comprehensive symptom profile, which aids in distinguishing IC/BPS from other conditions.

2. Commonly Used Assessment Scales and Questionnaires

The O'Leary-Sant Symptom and Problem Index (ICSI/ICPI)

Overview:

The O'Leary-Sant Symptom and Problem Index (ICSI/ICPI) is one of the most widely used questionnaires for evaluating IC/BPS. It consists of two separate indices: the Symptom Index (ICSI) and the Problem Index (ICPI).

- **ICSI:** Measures the frequency and severity of IC/BPS symptoms, including pain, urinary frequency, and urgency. It consists of questions rated on a scale from 0 to 4, where higher scores indicate greater symptom severity.

- **ICPI:** Assesses the degree to which IC/BPS symptoms interfere with daily life and activities. It also uses a scale from 0 to 4, with higher scores reflecting greater disruption to the patient's quality of life.

Administration:

- **Format:** The questionnaire is self-administered and typically completed by patients during clinical visits or as part of a research study.

- **Scoring:** Scores from the ICSI and ICPI are combined to provide an overall assessment of symptom severity and impact. Higher scores indicate more severe symptoms and greater impact on daily life.

Relevance:

- **Clinical Use:** The ICSI/ICPI is valuable for tracking symptom changes over time and evaluating treatment outcomes. It is frequently used in both clinical practice and research.

- **Limitations:** While comprehensive, it may not capture all aspects of the patient experience, particularly in cases with complex or atypical symptom profiles.

The Visual Analog Scale (VAS) for Pain

Overview:

The Visual Analog Scale (VAS) for pain is a simple and widely used tool for quantifying pain intensity. It involves a 10-cm line with endpoints labeled "no pain" and "worst possible pain."

- **Measurement:** Patients mark a point on the line that corresponds to their pain intensity, with the distance from the "no pain" end being measured in centimeters.
- **Scoring:** The score is the distance in centimeters from the left end of the line, providing a numerical value for pain intensity.

Administration:

- **Format:** The VAS can be administered in paper form or electronically. It is often used during clinical consultations or research assessments.
- **Frequency:** Patients may be asked to complete the VAS at regular intervals, such as before and after treatment, to monitor changes in pain levels.

Relevance:

- **Clinical Use:** The VAS is useful for assessing the intensity of pain associated with IC/BPS and evaluating the effectiveness of pain management strategies.
- **Limitations:** The VAS provides a single-dimensional measure of pain intensity and does not capture other pain-related factors, such as pain quality or impact on function.

The Bladder Pain Index (BPI)

Overview:

The Bladder Pain Index (BPI) is designed specifically to assess bladder pain and its impact on quality of life. It includes questions related to pain intensity, frequency of symptoms, and the overall impact on daily activities.

- **Components:** The BPI typically includes questions about pain intensity (rated on a scale), the frequency of pain episodes, and the effect of pain on daily functioning.

- **Scoring:** Scores are calculated based on the responses to each question, with higher scores indicating greater pain severity and impact.

Administration:

- **Format:** The BPI can be administered as a paper questionnaire or electronically. It is usually completed by patients during clinical evaluations or research studies.

- **Frequency:** It is often used at baseline and follow-up visits to assess changes in pain and its impact over time.

Relevance:

- **Clinical Use:** The BPI provides a comprehensive assessment of bladder pain and its consequences, helping clinicians tailor treatment plans to address specific pain-related issues.

- **Limitations:** The BPI focuses on bladder pain and may not capture other aspects of IC/BPS, such as urinary frequency or urgency.

The Interstitial Cystitis Impact Questionnaire (ICIQ)

Overview:

The Interstitial Cystitis Impact Questionnaire (ICIQ) is a tool used to evaluate the impact of IC/BPS on various aspects of the patient's life, including physical, emotional, and social domains.

- **Components:** The ICIQ includes questions about symptom frequency, pain, urinary frequency, and the impact of symptoms on daily activities and overall quality of life.
- **Scoring:** Responses are scored to provide a profile of the impact of IC/BPS on the patient's life, with higher scores indicating greater impact.

Administration:

- **Format:** The ICIQ is administered as a self-report questionnaire and can be completed on paper or electronically.
- **Frequency:** It is typically used at the start of treatment and during follow-up visits to monitor changes in the impact of IC/BPS.

Relevance:

- **Clinical Use:** The ICIQ helps clinicians understand how IC/BPS affects different areas of the patient's life, informing treatment decisions and patient counseling.
- **Limitations:** While comprehensive, the ICIQ may require additional assessment tools to capture all aspects of IC/BPS.

3. Benefits and Limitations of Assessment Tools

Benefits:

- **Standardization:** Assessment scales and questionnaires provide a standardized method for evaluating symptoms and their impact, ensuring consistency in clinical assessments and research.
- **Patient-Centered:** These tools capture the patient's perspective on symptoms and quality of life,

facilitating a more patient-centered approach to care.

- **Tracking Changes:** They enable clinicians to track changes in symptoms and quality of life over time, providing valuable information for adjusting treatment plans.

Limitations:

- **Subjectivity:** The subjective nature of self-report questionnaires may lead to variability in responses based on individual perceptions and interpretations of symptoms.

- **Complexity:** Some questionnaires may be lengthy or complex, potentially leading to patient fatigue or incomplete responses.

- **Cultural and Language Differences:** Variations in cultural and language backgrounds may affect how patients interpret and respond to questions, potentially impacting the accuracy of the results.

Conclusion

Assessment scales and questionnaires play a crucial role in the diagnosis, management, and monitoring of Interstitial Cystitis/Bladder Pain Syndrome (IC/BPS). Tools such as the O'Leary-Sant Symptom and Problem Index, Visual Analog Scale for pain, Bladder Pain Index, and Interstitial Cystitis Impact Questionnaire provide valuable insights into symptom severity, pain intensity, and quality of life. Each tool offers unique benefits and has specific limitations, making it essential for clinicians to use a combination of assessment methods to obtain a comprehensive understanding of the patient's condition. By integrating these tools into clinical practice, healthcare providers can enhance their ability to diagnose, manage, and treat IC/BPS effectively.

CHAPTER 4:
ETIOLOGY AND
PATHOPHYSIOLOGY

Theories of Interstitial Cystitis/Bladder Pain Syndrome (IC/BPS) Etiology

Interstitial Cystitis/Bladder Pain Syndrome (IC/BPS) is a complex and poorly understood condition characterized by chronic pelvic pain, urinary urgency, frequency, and discomfort. Despite extensive research, the exact etiology of IC/BPS remains elusive, and multiple theories have been proposed to explain its origins. This section explores the primary theories of IC/BPS etiology, including the roles of urothelial dysfunction, autoimmune and inflammatory processes, neurogenic factors, and genetic and environmental influences.

1. Urothelial Dysfunction Theory

Overview:

The urothelium is a specialized epithelial layer lining the bladder, playing a crucial role in maintaining the barrier function between the bladder lumen and the underlying tissue. Dysfunction of the urothelium has been proposed as a central factor in the development of IC/BPS.

- **Barrier Disruption:** One of the key hypotheses is that a defect in the urothelial barrier allows toxic substances from the urine to penetrate the bladder wall, leading to inflammation and pain. This barrier dysfunction can result from damage to the glycosaminoglycan (GAG) layer, a protective coating on the bladder surface.

- **Evidence:** Studies have shown that patients with IC/BPS often have reduced levels of GAGs in their bladder urine and a thinner GAG layer on the urothelium. This reduction can lead to increased permeability and potential exposure of the bladder wall to irritants.

- **Implications:** If urothelial dysfunction is a primary factor, therapies aimed at restoring the GAG layer or protecting the urothelium from irritants could be beneficial. This is supported by treatments such as bladder instillations with hyaluronic acid or chondroitin sulfate, which aim to replenish the GAG layer.

Limitations:

- Not all IC/BPS patients exhibit clear urothelial defects, and some patients with these defects do not have IC/BPS, suggesting that urothelial dysfunction alone may not account for all cases.

2. Autoimmune and Inflammatory Processes

Overview:

Autoimmune and inflammatory theories propose that IC/BPS results from an abnormal immune response leading to chronic inflammation in the bladder. This theory suggests that the body's immune system mistakenly targets bladder tissue, causing persistent inflammation and pain.

- **Autoimmune Response:** Some researchers believe that IC/BPS may be an autoimmune condition where the immune system attacks the bladder tissue. This theory is supported by the presence of inflammatory cells and cytokines in the bladder biopsies of IC/BPS patients.

- **Inflammatory Markers:** Elevated levels of pro-inflammatory cytokines, such as tumor necrosis factor-alpha (TNF-alpha) and interleukin-6 (IL-6), have been observed in the bladder and urine of IC/ BPS patients. These markers indicate an ongoing inflammatory process that may contribute to the symptoms of IC/BPS.

- **Hunner's Lesions:** The presence of Hunner's lesions, characterized by severe inflammation and ulceration in the bladder mucosa, supports the idea of an inflammatory component in IC/BPS. These lesions are often found in patients with Type 1 IC/BPS and are thought to result from a localized inflammatory response.

Limitations:

- While inflammation is evident in some patients, it is not present in all cases of IC/BPS, suggesting that other factors may contribute to the condition. Additionally, the exact cause of the inflammatory response remains unclear.

3. Neurogenic Factors

Overview:

The neurogenic theory posits that IC/BPS involves abnormalities in the nervous system, particularly the sensory nerves that innervate the bladder. According to this theory, altered nerve function or sensitization leads to heightened pain perception and bladder dysfunction.

- **Sensory Nerve Dysfunction:** Increased sensitivity or hyperactivity of sensory nerves in the bladder may result in the perception of pain and discomfort even in the absence of significant bladder pathology. This theory is supported by studies showing abnormal nerve growth and increased density of nerve fibers in the bladder wall of IC/BPS patients.

- **Pain Pathways:** Abnormalities in pain pathways,

including central sensitization, may contribute to the chronic pain experienced by IC/BPS patients. Central sensitization refers to an increased response to stimuli in the central nervous system, leading to heightened pain perception.

- **Neurogenic Bladder:** The concept of neurogenic bladder, where nerve damage or dysfunction leads to bladder symptoms, aligns with the neurogenic theory. Conditions such as interstitial cystitis with neurogenic bladder may overlap with IC/BPS.

Limitations:

- Neurogenic factors alone may not account for the full spectrum of IC/BPS symptoms. While nerve dysfunction is evident in some patients, it may be secondary to other underlying factors rather than a primary cause.

4. Genetic and Epigenetic Factors

Overview:

Genetic and epigenetic theories propose that genetic predisposition and epigenetic modifications play a role in the development of IC/BPS. These theories suggest that genetic variations and environmental interactions can influence susceptibility to the condition.

- **Genetic Predisposition:** Some studies have identified potential genetic markers associated with IC/BPS. Variations in genes related to inflammation, immune response, and bladder function may increase susceptibility to IC/BPS. Family history and genetic studies suggest a potential hereditary component in some cases.

- **Epigenetic Modifications:** Epigenetic changes, such as DNA methylation and histone modifications, can affect gene expression without altering the DNA sequence.

These modifications may influence susceptibility to IC/BPS by altering the expression of genes involved in inflammation, bladder function, and pain perception.

- **Environmental Interactions:** The interplay between genetic predisposition and environmental factors, such as infections, trauma, or exposure to irritants, may contribute to the development of IC/BPS. Epigenetic changes resulting from environmental exposures could influence the onset and progression of the condition.

Limitations:

- The genetic and epigenetic contributions to IC/BPS are complex and not fully understood. Identifying specific genetic markers and understanding their role in the development of IC/BPS remain areas of active research.

5. Other Theories

Overview:

In addition to the primary theories mentioned, other factors and theories have been proposed to explain IC/BPS etiology:

- **Bladder Microbiome:** Alterations in the bladder microbiome, or the community of microorganisms living in the bladder, have been explored as a potential factor in IC/BPS. Dysbiosis, or an imbalance in the microbiome, may contribute to bladder inflammation and symptoms.

- **Hormonal Influences:** Hormonal changes, particularly in women, may play a role in IC/BPS. Fluctuations in estrogen levels and other hormones have been associated with bladder symptoms, suggesting a hormonal component to the condition.

- **Psychosomatic Factors:** Psychological stress and psychosomatic factors may contribute to IC/BPS symptoms. Stress and emotional factors can influence pain perception and bladder function, potentially exacerbating symptoms.

Conclusion

The etiology of Interstitial Cystitis/Bladder Pain Syndrome (IC/BPS) is multifaceted and not fully understood. Theories such as urothelial dysfunction, autoimmune and inflammatory processes, neurogenic factors, and genetic and epigenetic influences offer valuable insights into potential causes and mechanisms underlying the condition. Each theory provides a piece of the puzzle, highlighting the complexity of IC/BPS and the need for a comprehensive approach to understanding and managing the condition.

Autoimmune and Allergic Mechanisms in Interstitial Cystitis/Bladder Pain Syndrome (IC/BPS)

Interstitial Cystitis/Bladder Pain Syndrome (IC/BPS) is a chronic condition characterized by pelvic pain, urinary urgency, and frequency. The precise etiology of IC/BPS remains unclear, but autoimmune and allergic mechanisms have emerged as significant areas of investigation. These mechanisms propose that IC/BPS may result from abnormal immune responses or hypersensitivity reactions leading to bladder inflammation and pain. This section explores the autoimmune and allergic theories in detail, examining their evidence, implications, and limitations.

1. Autoimmune Mechanisms

Overview:

Autoimmune mechanisms suggest that IC/BPS may be driven by an aberrant immune response in which the body's immune system mistakenly targets and damages bladder tissue. This theory posits that IC/BPS could be an autoimmune disorder where chronic inflammation results from immune-mediated damage.

Key Concepts:

- **Autoimmune Response:** The autoimmune theory implies that the immune system erroneously identifies bladder tissue as foreign, leading to chronic inflammation and tissue damage. This process can result in symptoms such as pain, urinary urgency, and frequency.

- **Autoantibodies and Immune Markers:** Evidence for autoimmune mechanisms includes the presence of autoantibodies and abnormal immune markers in some IC/BPS patients. For instance, autoantibodies against bladder tissue or components of the extracellular matrix have been detected. Elevated levels of pro-inflammatory cytokines and immune cells, such as T lymphocytes and macrophages, are also observed in the bladder wall of IC/BPS patients.

- **Hunner's Lesions:** The presence of Hunner's lesions, which are characterized by severe inflammation and ulceration of the bladder mucosa, is consistent with an autoimmune response. These lesions are found in Type 1 IC/BPS and may reflect localized autoimmune inflammation.

Evidence:

- **Histological Findings:** Biopsy studies of IC/BPS patients, particularly those with Hunner's lesions, reveal chronic inflammatory changes and immune cell infiltration. These findings support the notion of an autoimmune component in some cases of IC/BPS.

- **Response to Immunosuppressive Therapy:** Some patients with IC/BPS show improvement with immunosuppressive therapies, such as corticosteroids or immunomodulators. This response suggests that autoimmune mechanisms may play a role in the condition.

Limitations:

- **Variability in Autoimmune Markers:** Not all IC/BPS patients exhibit clear autoimmune markers, and autoimmune testing can be inconsistent. This variability suggests that autoimmune mechanisms may not be the sole factor in IC/BPS.

- **Overlap with Other Conditions:** Autoimmune features observed in IC/BPS patients may overlap with other autoimmune or inflammatory conditions, complicating the interpretation of these findings.

2. Allergic Mechanisms

Overview:

The allergic theory posits that IC/BPS could result from hypersensitivity reactions or allergic responses that lead to chronic inflammation and bladder symptoms. This theory suggests that environmental allergens or irritants may trigger an inappropriate immune response in the bladder.

Key Concepts:

- **Hypersensitivity Reactions:** Allergic mechanisms involve hypersensitivity reactions where the immune system overreacts to harmless substances, leading to inflammation and damage. In IC/BPS, allergens or irritants may provoke a hypersensitive response in the bladder.

- **Evidence of Allergic Response:** Some IC/BPS patients report an association between symptoms and exposure to certain foods, chemicals, or environmental factors, which may suggest an allergic component. Increased levels of histamine and other allergy-related mediators have been observed in some patients.

- **Bladder Mast Cells:** Mast cells are immune cells involved in allergic responses and are known to release histamine and other mediators that contribute to inflammation. Studies have found increased numbers of mast cells in the bladder wall of IC/BPS patients, which supports the role of allergic mechanisms.

Evidence:

- **Symptom Triggers:** Patients often identify specific triggers, such as certain foods or environmental allergens, that exacerbate their symptoms. This observation aligns with the allergic theory of IC/BPS.

- **Response to Antihistamines:** Some patients with IC/BPS experience relief from antihistamines or other allergy medications, suggesting that allergic or hypersensitivity mechanisms may play a role in their symptoms.

Limitations:

- **Non-Specific Findings:** The presence of mast cells and other allergy-related markers in IC/BPS patients is not exclusive to the condition. Mast cell activation and histamine release can occur in various other conditions, making it challenging to pinpoint an allergic mechanism.

- **Variability in Patient Response:** Not all IC/BPS patients show improvement with allergy treatments, indicating that allergic mechanisms may not be universally applicable.

3. Integrative Perspective

Overlap Between Autoimmune and Allergic Mechanisms:

Autoimmune and allergic mechanisms are not mutually exclusive and may overlap in the context of IC/BPS. For instance, a patient might exhibit both autoimmune features and allergic responses, with each contributing to the overall symptom profile. Understanding the interplay between these mechanisms can provide a more comprehensive view of IC/BPS pathogenesis.

Chronic Inflammation as a Common Link:

Both autoimmune and allergic theories highlight the role of chronic inflammation in IC/BPS. Whether driven by an autoimmune response, allergic reaction, or a combination of factors, persistent inflammation appears to be a common feature in the condition. Research into the underlying inflammatory pathways and immune responses may offer insights into more effective treatments.

4. Clinical Implications

Diagnostic Approaches:

- **Autoimmune Testing:** For patients suspected of having autoimmune IC/BPS, tests for autoantibodies and immune markers may be conducted. However, these tests should be interpreted in the context of other diagnostic findings.

- **Allergy Testing:** Patients with suspected allergic mechanisms may benefit from allergy testing to identify potential triggers. An elimination diet or avoidance of identified allergens may help manage symptoms.

Treatment Strategies:

- **Immunosuppressive Therapy:** For patients with evidence of autoimmune involvement, treatments such as corticosteroids or other immunomodulators may be considered. These therapies aim to reduce inflammation and modulate the immune response.

- **Antihistamines and Allergy Medications:** In cases where allergic mechanisms are suspected, antihistamines or other allergy medications may provide symptomatic relief. Addressing potential environmental or dietary triggers may also be beneficial.

Conclusion

Autoimmune and allergic mechanisms offer valuable perspectives on the etiology of Interstitial Cystitis/Bladder Pain Syndrome (IC/BPS). Autoimmune theories propose that IC/BPS may result from an aberrant immune response targeting bladder tissue, while allergic theories suggest that hypersensitivity reactions to environmental factors or allergens could play a role. Both theories emphasize the importance of chronic inflammation and provide insights into potential diagnostic and therapeutic approaches. Understanding these mechanisms, along with their limitations and the potential overlap between them, is crucial for developing effective strategies for managing and treating IC/BPS. Ongoing research is essential for elucidating the precise role of autoimmune and allergic factors in IC/BPS and improving patient outcomes.

Infectious and Post-Infectious Models in Interstitial Cystitis/ Bladder Pain Syndrome (IC/BPS)

Interstitial Cystitis/Bladder Pain Syndrome (IC/BPS) is a chronic condition characterized by pelvic pain, urinary urgency, and frequency. While the exact etiology remains unclear, infectious and post-infectious models have been proposed to explain the development of IC/BPS. These models suggest that infections or the aftermath of infections might play a significant role in the pathogenesis of IC/BPS. This section explores these models, including the evidence supporting them, their implications, and their limitations.

1. Infectious Models

Overview:

The infectious model proposes that IC/BPS may be triggered or exacerbated by bacterial or viral infections. According to this model, an infection can initiate an inflammatory response in the bladder that persists even after the infection is resolved, leading to chronic symptoms characteristic of IC/BPS.

Key Concepts:

- **Initial Infection:** The infectious model posits that an initial bacterial or viral infection can cause significant inflammation and damage to the bladder mucosa. Common pathogens considered in this model include uropathogenic E. coli, Chlamydia, and Mycoplasma.

- **Persistent Inflammation:** After the initial infection is cleared, chronic inflammation may persist due to immune dysregulation or tissue damage. This persistent inflammation can lead to ongoing symptoms such as pain, urgency, and frequency.

- **Biofilm Formation:** Some infectious agents, particularly uropathogenic bacteria, can form biofilms on the bladder mucosa. Biofilms are clusters of microorganisms embedded in a protective matrix that adhere to surfaces and are resistant to treatment. The presence of biofilms may contribute to chronic symptoms and make infections difficult to eradicate.

Evidence:

- **Increased Incidence of UTIs:** Studies have found that a significant number of IC/BPS patients report a history of recurrent urinary tract infections (UTIs) prior to the onset of symptoms. This association supports the idea that infections may play a role in IC/BPS development.

- **Pathogen Detection:** Research has detected bacterial DNA or antigens in the urine or bladder tissue of IC/BPS patients, suggesting a possible infectious etiology. However, these findings are not always consistent and do not establish causality.

- **Response to Antibiotics:** Some IC/BPS patients report

improvement with antibiotics, particularly those that target specific pathogens. This response supports the hypothesis that infections or bacterial components may contribute to IC/BPS symptoms.

Limitations:

- **Lack of Consistent Pathogen Identification:** Not all IC/BPS patients have detectable pathogens or respond to antibiotic therapy, indicating that infections may not be the sole cause of the condition.

- **Overlap with Other Conditions:** The presence of pathogens or biofilms in IC/BPS patients may also be found in individuals with other bladder conditions, complicating the interpretation of these findings.

2. Post-Infectious Models

Overview:

The post-infectious model suggests that IC/BPS may result from a sequela of a previous infection. According to this model, an initial infection can trigger a series of events leading to chronic bladder symptoms, even after the infection has been cleared.

Key Concepts:

- **Immune Response:** A post-infectious response involves a prolonged or aberrant immune reaction following the resolution of an infection. This response can lead to chronic inflammation, tissue damage, and sensitization of the bladder, resulting in IC/BPS symptoms.

- **Chronic Inflammation:** Following an infection, the immune system may continue to produce inflammatory mediators that persist long after the infection is gone. This persistent inflammation can cause ongoing symptoms and contribute to the development of IC/BPS.

- **Bladder Sensitization:** Repeated or severe infections can lead to sensitization of the bladder, making it more responsive to stimuli and more prone to pain and discomfort. Sensitized bladders may experience symptoms similar to those seen in IC/BPS.

Evidence:

- **Post-Infectious Symptoms:** Some IC/BPS patients report the onset of symptoms following a urinary tract infection or other types of infections. This temporal relationship supports the idea that post-infectious processes may contribute to IC/BPS.

- **Chronic Inflammation Markers:** Elevated levels of inflammatory cytokines and immune cells in the bladder of IC/BPS patients suggest a chronic inflammatory response that may be related to previous infections.

- **Treatment Response:** Some patients with IC/BPS show improvement with treatments that address chronic inflammation or modulate the immune response, supporting the post-infectious model.

Limitations:

- **Inconsistent Temporal Associations:** Not all IC/BPS patients have a clear history of preceding infections, and the timing and nature of post-infectious symptoms can vary widely.

- **Lack of Direct Evidence:** While the post-infectious model is supported by indirect evidence, direct evidence linking specific infections to IC/BPS development is limited. Further research is needed to establish a clear connection.

3. Integrative Perspective

Overlap Between Infectious and Post-Infectious Models:

The infectious and post-infectious models are not mutually exclusive and may overlap in the context of IC/BPS. For example, an initial infection may lead to both acute inflammation and long-term changes in bladder function and immune response. Understanding how these models interact can provide a more comprehensive view of IC/BPS pathogenesis.

Chronic Inflammation as a Common Feature:

Both models emphasize the role of chronic inflammation in IC/BPS. Whether triggered by an ongoing infection or a post-infectious immune response, persistent inflammation appears to be a common feature in the condition. Research into the underlying inflammatory pathways and their interaction with infections may offer insights into more effective treatments.

4. Clinical Implications

Diagnostic Approaches:

- **Infection Testing:** For patients with a suspected infectious component, testing for bacterial or viral pathogens may be conducted. Urine cultures, PCR assays, and bladder biopsies can help identify potential pathogens.

- **Post-Infectious Evaluation:** Patients with a history of infections should be evaluated for signs of chronic inflammation or immune dysregulation. Assessing inflammatory markers and immune responses may provide insights into post-infectious processes.

Treatment Strategies:

- **Antibiotic Therapy:** In cases where an infectious etiology is suspected, targeted antibiotic therapy may be used. However, it is important to consider the potential for antibiotic resistance and the need for careful evaluation of treatment response.

- **Anti-Inflammatory Therapy:** For patients with evidence of chronic inflammation or a post-infectious immune response, anti-inflammatory treatments may be beneficial. This includes medications such as corticosteroids, non-steroidal anti-inflammatory drugs (NSAIDs), or other immunomodulators.

Conclusion

Infectious and post-infectious models provide valuable perspectives on the etiology of Interstitial Cystitis/Bladder Pain Syndrome (IC/BPS). The infectious model suggests that initial infections can trigger chronic inflammation and symptoms, while the post-infectious model posits that immune responses following an infection may lead to persistent bladder symptoms. Both models highlight the role of chronic inflammation and offer insights into diagnostic and therapeutic approaches. Understanding the interplay between these models and their implications for IC/BPS pathogenesis is essential for developing effective treatments and improving patient outcomes. Ongoing research is crucial for elucidating the precise role of infections and post-infectious processes in IC/BPS and advancing our knowledge of this complex condition.

Neurogenic and Psychosomatic Factors in Interstitial Cystitis/Bladder Pain Syndrome (IC/BPS)

Interstitial Cystitis/Bladder Pain Syndrome (IC/BPS) is a chronic condition marked by pelvic pain, urinary urgency, and frequency. Its multifactorial nature makes it challenging to pinpoint a singular cause, but neurogenic and psychosomatic factors have gained significant attention in understanding the pathogenesis of IC/BPS. These factors highlight the complex interplay between the nervous system, psychological state, and physical symptoms. This section explores the role of neurogenic and psychosomatic factors in IC/BPS, examining evidence, implications, and limitations.

1. Neurogenic Factors

Overview:

Neurogenic factors refer to the influence of the nervous system on the development and persistence of IC/BPS symptoms. These factors involve abnormalities in nerve function, pain perception, and neural pathways that contribute to the chronic pain and discomfort experienced by IC/BPS patients.

Key Concepts:

- **Sensory Nerve Dysfunction:** In IC/BPS, sensory nerves in the bladder and pelvic region may become hyperactive or sensitized. This hyperexcitability can result in heightened pain perception and increased bladder sensitivity. Neurogenic inflammation, where nerve activation leads to inflammation and pain, is a key aspect of this dysfunction.

- **Central Sensitization:** Central sensitization refers to an increased sensitivity of the central nervous system (CNS) to stimuli. In IC/BPS, central sensitization can amplify pain signals, making patients more sensitive to pain and discomfort even in the absence of significant bladder pathology. This phenomenon involves changes in spinal cord and brain processing of pain.

- **Nerve Growth and Alterations:** Studies have found increased nerve density and altered nerve growth in the bladder wall of IC/BPS patients. Abnormalities in nerve fibers, including the presence of unmyelinated C fibers, are associated with heightened pain and discomfort.

Evidence:

- **Histological Findings:** Biopsy studies of IC/BPS patients often reveal increased nerve fibers and abnormal nerve growth in the bladder mucosa. These findings support the role of neurogenic factors in the pathogenesis of the condition.

- **Pain Modulation:** Patients with IC/BPS often exhibit altered pain modulation pathways, such as increased activation of pain-related brain regions. Functional imaging studies have shown changes in brain activity patterns associated with pain perception in these patients.

- **Treatment Response:** Some IC/BPS patients experience relief with treatments targeting nerve function or pain pathways, such as neuromodulation therapies or medications affecting neurotransmitter systems. This response suggests that neurogenic factors contribute to symptomatology.

Limitations:

- **Complex Interactions:** Neurogenic factors interact with other mechanisms, such as inflammation or autoimmune responses. Isolating the impact of neurogenic factors alone is challenging, and their role may vary among patients.

- **Variable Findings:** Not all IC/BPS patients exhibit clear neurogenic abnormalities, indicating that neurogenic factors may not account for the condition in every case.

2. Psychosomatic Factors

Overview:

Psychosomatic factors involve the interplay between psychological and physical aspects of health. In the context of IC/BPS, psychosomatic factors refer to how psychological stress, emotional well-being, and mental health may influence or exacerbate physical symptoms.

Key Concepts:

- **Stress and Symptom Exacerbation:** Psychological

stress and emotional distress can exacerbate IC/BPS symptoms by influencing pain perception and bladder function. Stress-induced changes in neurotransmitter levels, hormone regulation, and immune responses can contribute to symptom flare-ups.

- **Somatization:** Somatization refers to the manifestation of psychological distress as physical symptoms. IC/BPS patients with significant psychosomatic components may experience heightened pain or discomfort as a result of underlying emotional or psychological issues.

- **Coping Mechanisms:** Patients' coping mechanisms and psychological resilience can impact their experience of IC/BPS. Effective coping strategies may mitigate symptoms, while maladaptive coping mechanisms may exacerbate them.

Evidence:

- **Psychological Correlations:** Studies have found correlations between psychological factors, such as anxiety, depression, and stress, and the severity of IC/BPS symptoms. Patients with higher levels of psychological distress often report more intense pain and greater symptom burden.

- **Behavioral Interventions:** Behavioral therapies, such as cognitive-behavioral therapy (CBT) and stress management techniques, have shown benefits in reducing IC/BPS symptoms for some patients. These interventions aim to address psychological factors and improve coping strategies.

- **Quality of Life Impact:** IC/BPS significantly impacts patients' quality of life, including psychological well-being. Improved mental health and emotional support can lead to better overall management of the condition.

Limitations:

- **Complex Interactions:** The relationship between psychosomatic factors and IC/BPS symptoms is complex and bidirectional. Psychological distress can influence physical symptoms, but physical symptoms can also impact psychological well-being.

- **Individual Variability:** Not all IC/BPS patients have significant psychosomatic components. The influence of psychological factors may vary among individuals, and addressing these factors may not be sufficient for all patients.

3. Integrative Perspective

Overlap Between Neurogenic and Psychosomatic Factors:

Neurogenic and psychosomatic factors often intersect and influence each other in IC/BPS. For instance, psychological stress can exacerbate neurogenic inflammation and pain perception, while neurogenic abnormalities can influence psychological well-being. An integrative perspective considers how these factors interact and contribute to the overall symptomatology of IC/BPS.

Chronic Pain and Sensory Processing:

Both neurogenic and psychosomatic factors emphasize the role of chronic pain and altered sensory processing in IC/BPS. Chronic pain can lead to changes in neural pathways and psychological distress, creating a feedback loop that exacerbates symptoms.

4. Clinical Implications

Diagnostic Approaches:

- **Multidisciplinary Evaluation:** A comprehensive assessment of IC/BPS patients should include evaluation of both neurogenic and psychosomatic factors. This may involve neurological assessments, psychological evaluations, and consideration of stress and coping mechanisms.

- **Pain and Stress Assessment:** Tools to assess pain intensity, sensory processing, and psychological stress can help identify the contributions of neurogenic and psychosomatic factors to IC/BPS symptoms.

Treatment Strategies:

- **Neurogenic Treatments:** Therapies targeting neurogenic factors may include medications such as nerve relaxants, anticonvulsants, or neuromodulation techniques. These treatments aim to address nerve dysfunction and pain perception.

- **Psychosocial Interventions:** Addressing psychosomatic factors may involve behavioral therapies, stress management, and psychological support. Interventions such as cognitive-behavioral therapy (CBT) and mindfulness-based stress reduction (MBSR) can improve coping strategies and reduce symptom burden.

- **Integrated Approach:** Combining treatments that address both neurogenic and psychosomatic factors may provide a more comprehensive approach to managing IC/BPS. Coordinated care involving urologists, psychologists, and pain specialists can optimize patient outcomes.

Conclusion

Neurogenic and psychosomatic factors play significant roles in the pathogenesis and management of Interstitial Cystitis/ Bladder Pain Syndrome (IC/BPS). Neurogenic factors involve abnormalities in nerve function and pain perception, while psychosomatic factors encompass the influence of psychological stress and emotional well-being on physical symptoms. Understanding the interplay between these factors is crucial for developing effective diagnostic and treatment strategies. An integrative approach that addresses both neurogenic and psychosomatic components can improve patient outcomes and enhance overall management of IC/BPS. Ongoing research is essential for elucidating the complex interactions between these factors and advancing our knowledge of this challenging condition.

Interaction with Other Chronic Conditions in Interstitial Cystitis/Bladder Pain Syndrome (IC/BPS)

Interstitial Cystitis/Bladder Pain Syndrome (IC/BPS) is a complex and multifaceted disorder characterized by pelvic pain, urinary urgency, and frequency. The interplay between IC/BPS and other chronic conditions is a significant aspect of its clinical management. Understanding these interactions can provide insights into the underlying mechanisms of IC/BPS and guide more effective treatment strategies. This section explores the relationships between IC/BPS and other chronic conditions, including their impact on symptom presentation, disease management, and patient outcomes.

1. Comorbid Chronic Pain Conditions

Overview:

IC/BPS often coexists with other chronic pain conditions, such as fibromyalgia, irritable bowel syndrome (IBS), and chronic pelvic pain syndrome. The presence of multiple chronic pain conditions can complicate diagnosis and treatment, as symptoms may overlap and exacerbate each other.

Key Concepts:

- **Fibromyalgia:** Fibromyalgia is characterized by widespread musculoskeletal pain, fatigue, and tender points. Many patients with IC/BPS also experience symptoms of fibromyalgia, and both conditions share common features such as heightened pain sensitivity and central sensitization.

- **Irritable Bowel Syndrome (IBS):** IBS is a functional gastrointestinal disorder marked by abdominal pain, bloating, and altered bowel habits. Patients with IC/BPS frequently report IBS symptoms, and the two conditions often coexist. Shared mechanisms, such as increased visceral sensitivity and altered gut-brain interactions, may contribute to this overlap.

- **Chronic Pelvic Pain Syndrome:** Chronic pelvic pain syndrome (CPPS) encompasses a range of conditions affecting the pelvic region, including IC/BPS. The presence of CPPS can complicate the management of IC/BPS, as patients may have overlapping symptoms and require a multidisciplinary approach.

Evidence:

- **Symptom Overlap:** Studies have shown a high prevalence of comorbid chronic pain conditions in patients with IC/BPS. For instance, research indicates that 30-50% of IC/BPS patients also have fibromyalgia or IBS, highlighting the frequent coexistence of these disorders.

- **Shared Pathophysiology:** Common pathophysiological mechanisms, such as central sensitization and dysregulation of pain processing pathways, are present in both IC/BPS and other chronic pain conditions. These shared mechanisms contribute to symptom overlap and increased symptom burden.

- **Impact on Treatment:** The presence of comorbid chronic pain conditions can affect treatment efficacy and patient outcomes. Multimodal treatment approaches addressing both IC/BPS and comorbid conditions are often necessary for optimal management.

Limitations:

- **Complex Diagnosis:** The overlap of symptoms between IC/BPS and other chronic pain conditions can complicate diagnosis. Differentiating between primary IC/BPS symptoms and those attributable to comorbid conditions requires careful evaluation.

- **Varied Response to Treatment:** Treatment responses can vary based on the presence of comorbid conditions. Tailoring treatment strategies to address both IC/BPS and associated chronic pain conditions is essential for achieving optimal outcomes.

2. Autoimmune and Inflammatory Conditions

Overview:

IC/BPS may interact with autoimmune and inflammatory conditions, such as systemic lupus erythematosus (SLE), rheumatoid arthritis (RA), and inflammatory bowel disease (IBD). These interactions can influence the presentation and management of IC/BPS.

Key Concepts:

- **Systemic Lupus Erythematosus (SLE):** SLE is a systemic autoimmune disease characterized by widespread inflammation and organ involvement. Patients with SLE may experience IC/BPS symptoms as part of their disease spectrum, potentially due to autoimmune-mediated bladder inflammation.

- **Rheumatoid Arthritis (RA):** RA is an autoimmune condition primarily affecting the joints but can also involve systemic inflammation. The presence of RA may exacerbate IC/BPS symptoms through systemic inflammation and immune dysregulation.

- **Inflammatory Bowel Disease (IBD):** IBD, including Crohn's disease and ulcerative colitis, is characterized by chronic inflammation of the gastrointestinal tract.

The coexistence of IBD and IC/BPS may be related to shared inflammatory pathways and immune system dysregulation.

Evidence:

- **Prevalence of Comorbidities:** Research indicates that patients with IC/BPS may have a higher prevalence of autoimmune and inflammatory conditions compared to the general population. For example, studies have found increased rates of SLE and RA among IC/BPS patients.

- **Immune Dysregulation:** Shared immune dysregulation and inflammatory pathways between IC/BPS and autoimmune conditions suggest a potential link. Elevated levels of pro-inflammatory cytokines and immune cells are observed in both IC/BPS and autoimmune disorders.

- **Treatment Considerations:** The presence of autoimmune or inflammatory conditions can impact treatment choices for IC/BPS. Managing these comorbidities often requires a coordinated approach involving rheumatologists, gastroenterologists, and urologists.

Limitations:

- **Diagnostic Complexity:** The overlap of IC/BPS with autoimmune and inflammatory conditions can complicate diagnosis and management. Distinguishing between symptoms caused by IC/BPS and those related to comorbid conditions requires a comprehensive evaluation.

- **Therapeutic Challenges:** Treatments for autoimmune and inflammatory conditions may have interactions with therapies used for IC/BPS. Coordinated management is essential to address both conditions effectively.

3. Psychiatric and Psychological Conditions

Overview:

Psychiatric and psychological conditions, such as depression, anxiety, and post-traumatic stress disorder (PTSD), often coexist with IC/BPS. These conditions can affect symptom severity and overall quality of life.

Key Concepts:

- **Depression and Anxiety:** Depression and anxiety are common among IC/BPS patients and can exacerbate symptoms. Psychological distress can affect pain perception, coping mechanisms, and overall well-being.

- **Post-Traumatic Stress Disorder (PTSD):** PTSD, resulting from trauma or stress, may be associated with IC/BPS. The stress response and psychological trauma may contribute to the development or worsening of IC/BPS symptoms.

- **Impact on Quality of Life:** The presence of psychiatric and psychological conditions can significantly impact quality of life in IC/BPS patients. Addressing mental health concerns is crucial for comprehensive management.

Evidence:

- **Prevalence:** Studies have found high rates of depression, anxiety, and PTSD in IC/BPS patients. Research indicates that up to 50% of IC/BPS patients experience significant levels of psychological distress.

- **Correlation with Symptom Severity:** Psychological factors are often correlated with the severity of IC/BPS symptoms. Patients with higher levels of psychological distress tend to report more intense pain and greater functional impairment.

- **Benefits of Psychological Interventions:** Psychological interventions, such as cognitive-behavioral therapy (CBT) and mindfulness-based stress reduction (MBSR), have shown benefits in managing IC/BPS symptoms. These therapies can improve coping strategies and reduce psychological distress.

Limitations:

- **Bidirectional Influence:** The relationship between IC/BPS and psychiatric conditions is bidirectional. Psychological distress can worsen IC/BPS symptoms, while chronic pain and bladder issues can contribute to mental health problems.

- **Individual Variability:** The impact of psychiatric and psychological conditions on IC/BPS can vary among individuals. Tailoring mental health interventions to address specific needs is essential for effective management.

4. Integrative Perspective

Overlap and Interaction:

The interactions between IC/BPS and other chronic conditions underscore the importance of an integrative approach to diagnosis and treatment. The presence of comorbid conditions can complicate symptom management and require a multidisciplinary approach.

Comprehensive Care:

An integrative approach involves addressing both IC/BPS and comorbid conditions concurrently. Coordinated care involving specialists in urology, pain management, rheumatology, psychiatry, and other relevant fields is essential for optimizing patient outcomes.

5. Clinical Implications

Diagnostic Approaches:

- **Comprehensive Assessment:** A thorough evaluation of IC/BPS patients should include an assessment of comorbid chronic conditions. This may involve diagnostic tests, clinical interviews, and symptom questionnaires.

- **Multidisciplinary Collaboration:** Collaboration between healthcare providers across different specialties is crucial for managing IC/BPS and comorbid conditions. Coordinated care ensures that all aspects of the patient's health are addressed.

Treatment Strategies:

- **Tailored Treatment Plans:** Treatment plans should be individualized to address both IC/BPS and any comorbid conditions. Multimodal approaches that integrate pharmacological, behavioral, and lifestyle interventions are often necessary.

- **Integrated Therapies:** Combining therapies that address both IC/BPS and associated chronic conditions can improve overall outcomes. This may include medications, physical therapy, psychological support, and lifestyle modifications.

Conclusion

The interaction between Interstitial Cystitis/Bladder Pain Syndrome (IC/BPS) and other chronic conditions is a complex and multifaceted aspect of its management. Comorbid chronic pain conditions, autoimmune and inflammatory disorders, and psychiatric conditions can all influence IC/BPS symptoms and treatment strategies. An integrative approach that considers these interactions is essential for effective diagnosis and management. Coordinated care involving multidisciplinary teams and tailored treatment plans can optimize patient outcomes and improve quality of life. Ongoing research is crucial for further understanding the interplay between IC/BPS and comorbid conditions, enhancing our ability to address this challenging and multifactorial disorder.

CHAPTER 5: TREATMENT APPROACHES AND MANAGEMENT

Pharmacological Treatments for Interstitial Cystitis/Bladder Pain Syndrome (IC/BPS)

The management of Interstitial Cystitis/Bladder Pain Syndrome (IC/BPS) often requires a multifaceted approach, including pharmacological treatments. These treatments aim to alleviate pain, reduce inflammation, and improve bladder function. The pharmacological strategies can be categorized into several key areas: pain management, anti-inflammatory and immunomodulatory agents, bladder instillations, and antihistamines and mast cell stabilizers. This section provides an in-depth examination of these treatment modalities.

Pain Management: Analgesics and Antidepressants

Analgesics:

Analgesics are used to relieve pain and can be broadly classified into non-opioid and opioid categories.

- **Non-Opioid Analgesics:** Non-opioid analgesics, such as nonsteroidal anti-inflammatory drugs (NSAIDs) and acetaminophen, are often used as first-line treatments for pain in IC/BPS. NSAIDs, including ibuprofen and naproxen, work by inhibiting cyclooxygenase (COX) enzymes, reducing the synthesis of prostaglandins that mediate pain and inflammation. However, NSAIDs should be used with caution in patients with gastrointestinal or renal issues.

- **Acetaminophen:** Acetaminophen is a non-opioid analgesic that is often used for mild to moderate pain. It acts primarily in the central nervous system to reduce pain perception. While generally well-tolerated, it lacks anti-inflammatory properties and may not be as effective for inflammatory pain.

- **Opioids:** Opioid analgesics, such as oxycodone and hydrocodone, may be considered for severe pain unresponsive to non-opioid analgesics. Opioids work by binding to opioid receptors in the central nervous system, inhibiting pain transmission. Despite their effectiveness, opioids are associated with risks of dependence, tolerance, and adverse effects such as constipation and sedation.

Antidepressants:

Antidepressants are used not only for their effects on mood but also for their analgesic properties, particularly in chronic pain conditions like IC/BPS.

- **Tricyclic Antidepressants (TCAs):** TCAs, such as amitriptyline and nortriptyline, are commonly used in IC/BPS due to their analgesic effects. They work by increasing the levels of neurotransmitters such as serotonin and norepinephrine, which modulate pain pathways. TCAs can also have anticholinergic effects, which may contribute to their efficacy in managing bladder pain. Side effects include dry mouth, constipation, and blurred vision.

- **Selective Serotonin-Norepinephrine Reuptake Inhibitors (SNRIs):** SNRIs, such as duloxetine and venlafaxine, are another class of antidepressants used in the management of chronic pain. They act by inhibiting the reuptake of both serotonin and norepinephrine, which are involved in pain modulation. SNRIs may be preferred over TCAs in some patients due to a more favorable side effect profile.

- **Selective Serotonin Reuptake Inhibitors (SSRIs):** While SSRIs, such as sertraline and fluoxetine, are primarily used for mood disorders, they may also offer some benefit in pain management. They work by increasing serotonin levels, which can influence pain perception. However, their efficacy in IC/BPS is generally less pronounced compared to TCAs and SNRIs.

Anti-inflammatory and Immunomodulatory Agents

Anti-inflammatory Agents:

Anti-inflammatory medications are used to reduce inflammation, which may be a contributing factor in IC/BPS.

- **Nonsteroidal Anti-Inflammatory Drugs (NSAIDs):** As mentioned previously, NSAIDs such as ibuprofen and naproxen reduce inflammation by inhibiting COX enzymes and prostaglandin synthesis. They may provide symptomatic relief in IC/BPS, but their use is limited by potential gastrointestinal and renal side effects.

- **Corticosteroids:** Corticosteroids, such as prednisone, are powerful anti-inflammatory agents that can be used in severe cases of IC/BPS. They work by suppressing immune responses and reducing inflammation. Corticosteroids are generally used for short-term management due to potential side effects, including weight gain, hypertension, and immunosuppression.

Immunomodulatory Agents:

Immunomodulatory agents modify the immune response and may be used to manage IC/BPS with suspected autoimmune or inflammatory components.

- **Pentosan Polysulfate Sodium (PPS):** PPS is a polysulfated glycosaminoglycan used in the management of IC/BPS. It is believed to work by restoring the bladder's glycosaminoglycan (GAG) layer, which protects the bladder wall from irritants and reduces inflammation. Clinical trials have demonstrated its efficacy in improving symptoms and quality of life for IC/BPS patients.

- **Sodium Heparin:** Sodium heparin, an anticoagulant with anti-inflammatory properties, is sometimes used as a bladder instillation therapy. It may help reduce inflammation and pain by interfering with inflammatory pathways.

Bladder Instillations

Bladder instillations involve the direct administration of medications into the bladder via a catheter. This approach allows for targeted treatment and can be particularly useful for managing IC/BPS.

Common Bladder Instillations:

- **Dimethyl Sulfoxide (DMSO):** DMSO is a solvent with anti-inflammatory and analgesic properties. It is used as a bladder instillation to alleviate pain and inflammation in IC/BPS. DMSO is believed to work by reducing inflammation and acting as a local anesthetic. Its use is generally well-tolerated, but it may cause side effects such as bladder irritation or odor.

- **Hyaluronic Acid:** Hyaluronic acid is a component of the bladder's GAG layer and is used to replenish the protective mucosal layer. Instillation of hyaluronic acid can help restore the bladder lining and reduce symptoms. Clinical studies have shown its effectiveness in improving bladder function and reducing pain.

- **Heparin:** Bladder instillations with heparin can help reduce inflammation and pain by interfering with inflammatory processes. Heparin has been used in combination with other agents, such as corticosteroids, to enhance therapeutic outcomes.

Administration and Safety:

Bladder instillations are generally performed on an outpatient basis and require catheterization. The procedure is relatively safe, but potential risks include infection, bladder trauma, and discomfort during administration. Patients should be monitored for adverse effects and response to treatment.

Antihistamines and Mast Cell Stabilizers

Antihistamines:

Antihistamines are used to manage symptoms related to histamine release and mast cell activation, which are thought to play a role in IC/BPS.

- **H1-Receptor Antagonists:** H1-receptor antagonists, such as cetirizine and loratadine, are commonly used to alleviate allergy symptoms and may offer some benefit in IC/BPS. By blocking histamine receptors, these medications reduce histamine-mediated inflammation and irritation.

- **H2-Receptor Antagonists:** H2-receptor antagonists, like ranitidine, are primarily used to manage acid-related disorders but may also have some benefit in reducing histamine-induced bladder irritation. Their role in IC/BPS management is less well established compared to H1-receptor antagonists.

Mast Cell Stabilizers:

Mast cell stabilizers are used to prevent mast cell degranulation and reduce histamine release, which may be involved in IC/BPS.

- **Cromolyn Sodium:** Cromolyn sodium is a mast cell stabilizer used to prevent the release of histamine and other inflammatory mediators from mast cells. It is used as a bladder instillation in IC/BPS to reduce symptoms related to mast cell activation. While effective for some patients, its use is limited by the need for regular administration and potential side effects such as local irritation.

- **Ketotifen:** Ketotifen is an oral mast cell stabilizer with antihistaminic properties. It is used to manage allergy symptoms and may also have a role in managing IC/BPS symptoms. It works by stabilizing mast cells and reducing the release of inflammatory mediators.

Efficacy and Considerations:

The efficacy of antihistamines and mast cell stabilizers in IC/BPS varies among patients. While these agents may provide symptomatic relief for some, their benefits are not universally experienced. Individual response and tolerability should guide their use in IC/BPS management.

Conclusion

Pharmacological treatments for Interstitial Cystitis/Bladder Pain Syndrome (IC/BPS) encompass a range of medications aimed at managing pain, reducing inflammation, and improving bladder function. Analgesics, antidepressants, anti-inflammatory agents, bladder instillations, and antihistamines/ mast cell stabilizers each play a role in addressing different aspects of the condition. Effective management often requires a combination of these therapies, tailored to the individual patient's needs and response to treatment. Ongoing evaluation and adjustment of treatment strategies are essential for optimizing outcomes and improving quality of life for IC/BPS patients.

Non-Pharmacological Therapies for Interstitial Cystitis/ Bladder Pain Syndrome (IC/BPS)

In the management of Interstitial Cystitis/Bladder Pain Syndrome (IC/BPS), non-pharmacological therapies play a crucial role in complementing pharmacological treatments and addressing symptoms from multiple angles. These therapies encompass physical therapy and pelvic floor rehabilitation, dietary modifications and nutritional supplements, behavioral therapies and cognitive-behavioral therapy, as well as alternative and complementary medicine. Each of these approaches offers unique benefits and can contribute significantly to improving patient outcomes and quality of life.

Physical Therapy and Pelvic Floor Rehabilitation

Physical Therapy:

Physical therapy is a cornerstone in the non-pharmacological management of IC/BPS, particularly when pelvic floor dysfunction contributes to symptoms. Physical therapy focuses on strengthening and relaxing the muscles of the pelvic floor, improving bladder function, and reducing pain.

- **Pelvic Floor Exercises:** Pelvic floor exercises, including Kegel exercises, are designed to strengthen the muscles that support the bladder and pelvic organs. For IC/BPS patients, these exercises can help improve bladder control and reduce symptoms by enhancing muscle tone and endurance. A physical therapist can guide patients in proper technique and progression.

- **Manual Therapy:** Manual therapy involves hands-on techniques to alleviate pain and dysfunction. Techniques such as myofascial release, trigger point therapy, and deep tissue massage can be used to release tension and improve muscle function in the pelvic floor and surrounding areas. These methods may help alleviate pain and improve comfort.

- **Biofeedback:** Biofeedback is a technique that provides real-time feedback on physiological functions, allowing patients to gain control over their pelvic floor muscles. Through visual or auditory cues, patients learn to recognize and modify muscle contractions. Biofeedback can help patients improve muscle coordination and reduce pain associated with IC/BPS.

Pelvic Floor Rehabilitation:

Pelvic floor rehabilitation is a specialized form of physical therapy focusing on the pelvic floor muscles, ligaments, and connective tissues. It aims to address dysfunctions that may contribute to IC/BPS symptoms.

- **Assessment and Diagnosis:** A thorough assessment by a pelvic floor specialist includes evaluating muscle strength, flexibility, and coordination. This assessment helps identify specific dysfunctions and guides the development of an individualized treatment plan.

- **Stretching and Relaxation Techniques:** Techniques such as stretching and relaxation exercises help relieve muscle tension and improve flexibility. These methods are particularly beneficial for patients with muscle tightness or spasms in the pelvic floor.

- **Education and Lifestyle Modifications:** Pelvic floor rehabilitation often includes education on lifestyle modifications, posture, and body mechanics. Patients may be advised on strategies to minimize strain on the pelvic floor and improve overall function.

Evidence and Efficacy:

- **Clinical Studies:** Research supports the efficacy of physical therapy and pelvic floor rehabilitation in managing IC/BPS. Studies have shown improvements in pain, bladder symptoms, and quality of life with targeted physical therapy interventions.

- **Patient Outcomes:** Many patients report significant benefits from physical therapy, including reduced pain, improved bladder control, and enhanced overall function. Regular participation in physical therapy and adherence to prescribed exercises contribute to positive outcomes.

Limitations:

- **Individual Variation:** The effectiveness of physical therapy can vary based on individual factors, including the presence of comorbid conditions and the severity of IC/BPS symptoms. A personalized approach is essential for optimal results.

- **Duration and Commitment:** Physical therapy often requires ongoing sessions and patient commitment. Adherence to home exercises and lifestyle modifications is crucial for achieving long-term benefits.

Dietary Modifications and Nutritional Supplements

Dietary Modifications:

Dietary modifications can play a significant role in managing IC/BPS symptoms. Certain foods and beverages may exacerbate symptoms, while others can help alleviate discomfort.

- **Elimination Diet:** An elimination diet involves removing potentially irritating foods and beverages from the diet to identify triggers. Common irritants include caffeine, alcohol, spicy foods, acidic foods (e.g., citrus fruits), and artificial sweeteners. Patients reintroduce these foods gradually to assess their impact on symptoms.

- **Bladder-Friendly Diet:** A bladder-friendly diet emphasizes foods that are less likely to irritate the bladder. Recommendations may include increasing the intake of non-acidic fruits, vegetables, whole grains, and lean proteins. Hydration is also important, with an emphasis on drinking adequate water and avoiding excessive caffeine and alcohol.

Nutritional Supplements:

Nutritional supplements may be used to support overall health and address specific deficiencies or imbalances that could affect IC/BPS symptoms.

- **Pentosan Polysulfate Sodium (PPS):** PPS is a glycosaminoglycan that is believed to help restore the bladder's protective layer. It is used as both a supplement and a bladder instillation in the management of IC/BPS. Clinical evidence supports its efficacy in improving symptoms and quality of life.

- **Omega-3 Fatty Acids:** Omega-3 fatty acids, found in fish oil and flaxseed oil, have anti-inflammatory properties. Supplementation with omega-3s may help reduce inflammation and improve overall bladder health.

- **Probiotics:** Probiotics are beneficial bacteria that support gut health and may have an impact on systemic inflammation. While evidence is limited, some patients with IC/BPS may benefit from probiotics as part of a comprehensive approach to managing symptoms.

Evidence and Efficacy:

- **Dietary Studies:** Research has shown that dietary modifications can lead to improvements in IC/BPS symptoms. Patients who identify and avoid personal triggers often experience symptom relief.

- **Supplemental Research:** Evidence supporting the use of nutritional supplements is varied. While some supplements, such as PPS, have demonstrated efficacy in clinical trials, others require further research to establish their role in IC/BPS management.

Limitations:

- **Individual Variation:** The impact of dietary modifications and supplements can vary widely among individuals. Personalization of dietary recommendations is essential for addressing specific triggers and nutritional needs.

- **Potential Interactions:** Supplements can interact with medications and other treatments. Patients should consult with healthcare providers before starting new supplements to ensure safety and avoid adverse effects.

Behavioral Therapies and Cognitive-Behavioral Therapy

Behavioral Therapies:

Behavioral therapies focus on modifying behavior and thought patterns to manage pain and improve quality of life. These therapies are based on the understanding that psychological factors can influence the perception and management of pain.

- **Biofeedback Therapy:** Biofeedback therapy involves using electronic devices to provide real-time feedback on physiological functions, such as muscle tension and heart rate. Patients learn to control these functions through relaxation and visualization techniques. Biofeedback can help manage pain and reduce stress associated with IC/BPS.

- **Relaxation Techniques:** Relaxation techniques, such as deep breathing exercises, progressive muscle relaxation, and guided imagery, help reduce stress and promote overall well-being. These techniques can be integrated into daily routines to manage symptoms and improve coping strategies.

Cognitive-Behavioral Therapy (CBT):

Cognitive-behavioral therapy (CBT) is a structured, goal-oriented therapy that addresses negative thought patterns and behaviors contributing to pain and distress. CBT for IC/BPS focuses on improving coping strategies and reducing the impact of symptoms on daily life.

- **Cognitive Restructuring:** Cognitive restructuring involves identifying and challenging negative thought patterns that contribute to pain and discomfort. Patients learn to reframe their thoughts and develop more positive and adaptive ways of thinking.

- **Behavioral Activation:** Behavioral activation encourages patients to engage in meaningful and enjoyable activities despite pain. This approach helps counteract feelings of depression and inactivity, promoting a more active and fulfilling life.

- **Stress Management:** CBT includes stress management techniques to help patients cope with the emotional and psychological aspects of IC/BPS. Techniques may include relaxation exercises, time management strategies, and problem-solving skills.

Evidence and Efficacy:

- **Clinical Trials:** Research supports the effectiveness of behavioral therapies and CBT in managing chronic pain conditions, including IC/BPS. Studies have shown improvements in pain levels, quality of life, and psychological well-being with these approaches.

- **Patient Reports:** Many patients report significant benefits from behavioral therapies and CBT, including reduced pain perception, improved coping skills, and enhanced overall well-being.

Limitations:

- **Access to Therapy:** Access to qualified therapists and CBT programs may be limited in some areas. Patients may need to seek out specialized services or online resources to access these therapies.

- **Individual Response:** The effectiveness of behavioral therapies and CBT can vary among individuals. Personalization of therapy and ongoing support are essential for achieving optimal results.

Alternative and Complementary Medicine

Acupuncture:

Acupuncture is an alternative therapy that involves inserting thin needles into specific points on the body to stimulate energy flow and promote healing. In the context of IC/BPS, acupuncture is believed to help manage pain and improve bladder function.

- **Mechanism of Action:** Acupuncture is thought to work by stimulating the release of endorphins and modulating pain pathways. It may also improve blood flow and reduce inflammation.

- **Clinical Evidence:** Research on the efficacy of acupuncture for IC/BPS is limited but suggests potential benefits for pain relief and symptom management. More rigorous studies are needed to confirm its effectiveness.

Herbal Medicine:

Herbal medicine involves using plant-based substances to support health and manage symptoms. Several herbs have been explored for their potential benefits in IC/BPS.

- **Corn Silk:** Corn silk (Zea mays) has been used traditionally for urinary tract issues. It is believed to have anti-inflammatory and soothing properties that may help alleviate IC/BPS symptoms.

- **Marshmallow Root:** Marshmallow root (Althaea officinalis) is another herb with demulcent properties. It may help soothe and protect the bladder lining, potentially reducing irritation and pain.

- **Clinical Evidence:** Evidence supporting the use of herbal medicine for IC/BPS is limited and often based on traditional use. Patients should consult with healthcare providers before using herbal remedies to ensure safety and avoid potential interactions.

Mind-Body Therapies:

Mind-body therapies focus on the connection between mental and physical health. Techniques such as mindfulness meditation, yoga, and tai chi are used to promote relaxation and reduce stress.

- **Mindfulness Meditation:** Mindfulness meditation involves focusing on the present moment and accepting thoughts and feelings without judgment. It can help manage pain and reduce stress associated with IC/BPS.

- **Yoga:** Yoga combines physical postures, breathing exercises, and meditation to promote relaxation and flexibility. Yoga may help alleviate pain, improve bladder function, and enhance overall well-being.

- **Tai Chi:** Tai chi is a gentle martial art that involves slow, flowing movements and deep breathing. It has been shown to improve physical function and reduce stress, which may benefit IC/BPS patients.

Evidence and Efficacy:

- **Research and Patient Reports:** Studies on alternative and complementary medicine for IC/BPS are limited but suggest potential benefits in managing symptoms and improving quality of life. Patient reports and anecdotal evidence often highlight positive outcomes.

- **Integration with Conventional Care:** Many patients find value in integrating alternative and complementary therapies with conventional medical treatments. Collaboration with healthcare providers ensures a comprehensive approach to symptom management.

Limitations:

- **Lack of Standardization:** Alternative and complementary therapies can lack standardization and regulation, leading to variability in quality and efficacy. Patients should seek reputable practitioners and evidence-based approaches.

- **Potential Interactions:** Some alternative therapies may interact with conventional treatments or have side effects. Consultation with healthcare providers is essential to ensure safe and effective use.

Conclusion

Non-pharmacological therapies play a vital role in the comprehensive management of Interstitial Cystitis/Bladder Pain Syndrome (IC/BPS). Physical therapy and pelvic floor rehabilitation address musculoskeletal and functional aspects, while dietary modifications and nutritional supplements help manage potential triggers and support overall health. Behavioral therapies and cognitive-behavioral therapy provide strategies for managing pain and improving coping skills, and alternative and complementary medicine offers additional options for symptom relief. Integrating these approaches with conventional treatments can enhance patient outcomes and quality of life, emphasizing the importance of a holistic and individualized approach to managing IC/BPS.

Interventional and Surgical Options for Interstitial Cystitis/ Bladder Pain Syndrome (IC/BPS)

Interventional and surgical treatments are considered when non-pharmacological and pharmacological approaches fail to provide adequate relief for patients with Interstitial Cystitis/ Bladder Pain Syndrome (IC/BPS). These options aim to improve symptoms, restore bladder function, and enhance quality of life. This section explores three major interventional and surgical options: bladder hydrodistention, neuromodulation techniques, and surgical procedures such as cystectomy and augmentation cystoplasty.

Bladder Hydrodistention

Bladder Hydrodistention Overview:

Bladder hydrodistention, also known as hydrodistention, is a minimally invasive procedure used to manage IC/BPS symptoms. The procedure involves the inflation of the bladder with fluid to stretch the bladder walls and potentially reduce symptoms.

- **Procedure Details:** During the procedure, the patient is placed under general or regional anesthesia. A cystoscope is inserted through the urethra to visualize the bladder. Sterile fluid, usually saline or a sterile solution, is then slowly infused into the bladder. The bladder is distended to a specific pressure and volume, and the fluid is retained for a few minutes before being drained.

- **Mechanism of Action:** The exact mechanism by which bladder hydrodistention alleviates symptoms is not fully understood. The procedure may work by stretching the bladder wall, disrupting pain pathways, or altering the bladder's sensory perception. It may also help by increasing the bladder's capacity and improving bladder function.

Efficacy and Evidence:

- **Clinical Studies:** Several studies have demonstrated

the efficacy of bladder hydrodistention in providing symptomatic relief for IC/BPS patients. Research indicates that many patients experience significant improvement in pain and bladder function following the procedure. However, the duration of symptom relief can vary, and some patients may require multiple treatments.

- **Patient Reports:** Patients often report temporary relief of symptoms following bladder hydrodistention. The procedure can be effective in reducing pain, urinary frequency, and urgency. However, the effects may be short-lived for some patients, necessitating repeated treatments.

Risks and Complications:

- **Potential Risks:** Bladder hydrodistention is generally safe, but potential risks include infection, bleeding, bladder perforation, and transient worsening of symptoms. Some patients may experience discomfort or pain during and after the procedure.

- **Post-Procedure Care:** Patients may need to follow specific post-procedure instructions, including avoiding strenuous activities and monitoring for signs of infection. Pain management and bladder training exercises may also be recommended to enhance recovery and maintain symptom relief.

Neuromodulation Techniques

Neuromodulation Overview:

Neuromodulation techniques involve the use of electrical impulses to modulate nerve activity and influence bladder function. These techniques are used to manage IC/BPS symptoms by altering abnormal nerve signals and improving bladder control.

- **Sacral Neuromodulation (SNM):** Sacral

neuromodulation is a common neuromodulation technique used to manage IC/BPS. The procedure involves the implantation of a small device that delivers electrical impulses to the sacral nerves, which control bladder function.

- **Procedure Details:** A small electrode is implanted near the sacral nerves, typically in the lower back area. An external pulse generator is initially used to test the device's efficacy before permanent implantation. If successful, a permanent pulse generator is implanted under the skin, and the electrode remains in place.

- **Mechanism of Action:** Sacral neuromodulation works by stimulating the sacral nerves to modulate nerve activity and improve bladder function. It may help reduce symptoms such as pain, urgency, and frequency by altering abnormal nerve signals and restoring normal bladder activity.

- **Efficacy and Evidence:** Clinical studies have shown that sacral neuromodulation can be effective in reducing IC/BPS symptoms and improving quality of life. Many patients experience significant symptom relief and enhanced bladder control. The procedure is considered a viable option for patients who do not respond to conservative treatments.

- **Risks and Complications:** Risks of sacral neuromodulation include infection, device-related complications, and inadequate response to therapy. Some patients may experience discomfort at the implantation site or changes in sensory perception.

- **Percutaneous Tibial Nerve Stimulation (PTNS):** Percutaneous tibial nerve stimulation is a less invasive neuromodulation technique that involves stimulating the tibial nerve, which indirectly affects the sacral nerves responsible for bladder control.

- **Procedure Details:** PTNS is performed on an outpatient basis. A thin needle electrode is inserted near the tibial nerve in the ankle, and electrical impulses are delivered to stimulate the nerve. Treatment typically involves a series of sessions over several weeks.

- **Mechanism of Action:** PTNS works by modulating nerve activity through indirect stimulation of the sacral nerves. It aims to improve bladder function and reduce symptoms of IC/BPS by altering abnormal nerve signals.

- **Efficacy and Evidence:** Studies have shown that PTNS can provide symptomatic relief for IC/BPS patients, including reductions in pain, frequency, and urgency. The procedure is less invasive compared to sacral neuromodulation and may be a suitable option for patients seeking a less invasive approach.

- **Risks and Complications:** PTNS is generally well-tolerated, with minimal risks. Potential side effects include localized pain, bruising, or infection at the needle insertion site.

Surgical Procedures: Cystectomy and Augmentation Cystoplasty

Cystectomy:

Cystectomy is a surgical procedure involving the removal of all or part of the bladder. It is considered for patients with severe IC/BPS who do not respond to other treatments and have significant impairment of bladder function.

- **Types of Cystectomy:**
  - **Partial Cystectomy:** Involves the removal of a

portion of the bladder. This procedure may be considered for patients with localized bladder issues but is less common for IC/BPS.

- **Total Cystectomy:** Involves the complete removal of the bladder. This procedure is reserved for patients with severe, refractory IC/BPS. After total cystectomy, a urinary diversion is required to allow urine to exit the body.

- **Procedure Details:** Cystectomy is performed under general anesthesia. The procedure involves removing the bladder through an incision in the abdomen. After bladder removal, a urinary diversion is created, which can involve constructing a new bladder (neobladder), creating a conduit for urine to exit the body, or using an internal pouch.

- **Mechanism of Action:** The goal of cystectomy is to alleviate severe symptoms by removing the source of pain and dysfunction. Urinary diversion methods ensure continued urine elimination and aim to provide functional and quality-of-life improvements.

- **Efficacy and Evidence:** Cystectomy can provide significant relief for patients with severe IC/BPS who do not respond to other treatments. The procedure often results in improved quality of life and symptom relief. However, it is a major surgery with potential risks and complications.

- **Risks and Complications:** Risks include surgical complications, infection, urinary diversion-related issues, and changes in sexual function. Post-operative care and long-term follow-up are essential to address complications and manage the new urinary diversion.

Augmentation Cystoplasty:

Augmentation cystoplasty is a surgical procedure used to

increase bladder capacity and improve bladder function. It involves enlarging the bladder using a segment of bowel or other tissue.

- **Procedure Details:** During augmentation cystoplasty, a section of the bowel (usually the ileum or colon) is removed and used to augment the bladder. The bowel segment is attached to the bladder, increasing its capacity and allowing for improved storage of urine.

- **Mechanism of Action:** The procedure aims to alleviate symptoms of IC/BPS by increasing bladder capacity and reducing urinary frequency and urgency. The augmented bladder can accommodate more urine, leading to fewer episodes of discomfort and improved bladder function.

- **Efficacy and Evidence:** Augmentation cystoplasty has been shown to improve bladder capacity and reduce symptoms in patients with severe IC/BPS. Clinical studies and patient reports indicate significant improvements in bladder function and quality of life following the procedure.

- **Risks and Complications:** Risks include surgical complications, infection, bowel-related issues, and changes in bladder function. Patients may also experience complications related to the bowel segment used for augmentation. Long-term follow-up is necessary to monitor for potential issues and ensure optimal outcomes.

Conclusion

Interventional and surgical options for Interstitial Cystitis/ Bladder Pain Syndrome (IC/BPS) provide important alternatives for patients who do not achieve adequate relief through conservative treatments. Bladder hydrodistention offers a minimally invasive approach to symptom management, while neuromodulation techniques such as sacral neuromodulation and percutaneous tibial nerve stimulation offer targeted modulation of nerve activity. Surgical options, including cystectomy and augmentation cystoplasty, are considered for patients with severe, refractory symptoms and aim to provide substantial symptom relief and improved bladder function. Each of these approaches has its own benefits, risks, and considerations, and a personalized treatment plan should be developed in consultation with healthcare providers to address individual patient needs and optimize outcomes.

CHAPTER 6: PROGNOSIS AND OUTCOMES

Long-Term Management and Follow-Up for Interstitial Cystitis/Bladder Pain Syndrome (IC/BPS)

Long-term management and follow-up for Interstitial Cystitis/ Bladder Pain Syndrome (IC/BPS) are critical components of comprehensive care aimed at optimizing patient outcomes and enhancing quality of life. Due to the chronic and often unpredictable nature of IC/BPS, a multifaceted approach that includes ongoing assessment, individualized treatment adjustments, and patient education is essential. This section explores the key elements of long-term management and follow-up for IC/BPS, including monitoring, treatment adjustments, patient self-management, and coordination of care.

Monitoring and Regular Assessment

Objective: Regular monitoring and assessment are vital to evaluate the effectiveness of treatments, track symptom progression, and identify potential complications.

- **Scheduled Follow-Up Appointments:** Patients with IC/BPS should have regular follow-up appointments with their healthcare provider to assess symptom control, treatment efficacy, and any side effects or complications. The frequency of visits may vary based on the severity of symptoms and the treatment regimen.

- **Symptom Tracking:** Healthcare providers often use symptom diaries or questionnaires to track the frequency, intensity, and impact of IC/BPS symptoms. These tools help assess changes in symptoms over time and guide treatment adjustments.

- **Functional Assessments:** Regular assessments of bladder function, including urodynamic studies, may be performed to evaluate bladder capacity, compliance, and detrusor function. These assessments help determine the effectiveness of interventions and guide further management.

- **Quality of Life Evaluations:** Patient-reported outcomes related to quality of life, such as pain levels, urinary frequency, and overall well-being, are crucial for understanding the impact of IC/BPS on daily life. Tools like the Interstitial Cystitis Symptom Index (ICSI) and the Patient-Reported Outcomes Measurement Information System (PROMIS) may be used for this purpose.

Treatment Adjustments and Optimization

Objective: Treatment adjustments are necessary to address changes in symptoms, response to therapy, and emerging side effects.

- **Reviewing Treatment Efficacy:** During follow-up visits, healthcare providers should review the effectiveness of current treatments, including medications, physical therapy, and other interventions. Adjustments may be made based on symptom control and patient feedback.

- **Medication Management:** For patients on pharmacological treatments, regular evaluation of medication efficacy and side effects is important. Dose adjustments, switching medications, or combining therapies may be necessary to achieve optimal symptom management.

· **Non-Pharmacological Interventions:** Evaluating the effectiveness of non-pharmacological therapies, such as physical therapy and dietary modifications, is also important. Adjustments to these interventions may be required based on patient progress and evolving needs.

· **Interventional and Surgical Options:** For patients who have undergone interventional or surgical procedures, ongoing assessment of outcomes and potential complications is essential. Follow-up care should include monitoring for any adverse effects and assessing the long-term benefits of these interventions.

Patient Self-Management and Education

Objective: Empowering patients with knowledge and skills for self-management can improve adherence to treatment plans and overall outcomes.

· **Patient Education:** Providing comprehensive education about IC/BPS, including its nature, treatment options, and management strategies, is crucial. Patients should understand their condition, potential triggers, and how to manage symptoms effectively.

· **Self-Care Strategies:** Patients should be educated on self-care techniques, such as bladder training, pelvic floor exercises, and stress management. Training in using symptom diaries and tracking tools can help patients monitor their condition and make informed decisions about their care.

· **Lifestyle Modifications:** Guidance on lifestyle modifications, including dietary changes and activity levels, can help manage symptoms and improve overall health. Patients should be informed about bladder-friendly diets, hydration strategies, and the impact of stress on their condition.

- **Support Resources:** Connecting patients with support groups, counseling services, and online resources can provide additional support and encouragement. Peer support and shared experiences can be valuable in coping with the challenges of IC/BPS.

Coordination of Care and Multidisciplinary Approach

Objective: A multidisciplinary approach ensures that all aspects of a patient's care are addressed and coordinated effectively.

- **Multidisciplinary Team:** Managing IC/BPS often involves collaboration among various healthcare professionals, including urologists, pain specialists, physical therapists, dietitians, and mental health professionals. A coordinated approach ensures comprehensive care and addresses the diverse needs of patients.

- **Communication and Collaboration:** Effective communication among healthcare providers is essential for coordinating care and ensuring that treatment plans are aligned. Regular case reviews and interdisciplinary meetings can facilitate this process.

- **Patient-Centered Care:** A patient-centered approach involves tailoring treatment plans to individual needs and preferences. Involving patients in decision-making and setting goals for their care can enhance engagement and adherence to treatment plans.

Addressing Long-Term Challenges and Complications

Objective: Identifying and managing long-term challenges and complications is essential for maintaining quality of life and preventing adverse outcomes.

- **Managing Chronic Pain:** For patients with persistent pain despite treatment, ongoing pain management strategies should be employed. This may include adjustments to pain medications, exploring alternative therapies, and addressing psychosocial aspects of pain.

- **Bladder Function Monitoring:** Long-term monitoring of bladder function is important for detecting changes or complications related to bladder capacity, compliance, or function. Regular assessments can help manage issues such as decreased bladder capacity or detrusor overactivity.

- **Complications from Interventions:** Patients who have undergone surgical or interventional procedures may experience complications such as infection, device-related issues, or changes in urinary function. Regular follow-up is necessary to address these complications and provide appropriate interventions.

- **Psychosocial Support:** Chronic conditions like IC/BPS can impact mental health and emotional well-being. Providing access to mental health support and counseling can help patients cope with the psychological aspects of their condition.

Future Directions and Research

Objective: Staying informed about emerging treatments and research advancements can improve long-term management and care strategies.

- **Ongoing Research:** Research into the causes, pathophysiology, and treatment of IC/BPS is continually evolving. Staying updated on new findings and emerging therapies can inform treatment strategies and provide patients with the latest options.

- **Clinical Trials:** Participation in clinical trials may

offer access to innovative treatments and contribute to advancing knowledge about IC/BPS. Patients should be informed about available trials and the potential benefits and risks of participation.

- **Advancements in Technology:** Advances in medical technology, such as new diagnostic tools and treatment modalities, may enhance the management of IC/BPS. Keeping abreast of technological developments can improve patient care and outcomes.

Conclusion

Long-term management and follow-up for Interstitial Cystitis/ Bladder Pain Syndrome (IC/BPS) are essential for optimizing patient outcomes and enhancing quality of life. Regular monitoring and assessment, treatment adjustments, patient self-management, and a multidisciplinary approach are key components of effective care. Addressing long-term challenges and complications, staying informed about research advancements, and coordinating care with a patient-centered focus can significantly impact the management of IC/BPS. By providing comprehensive, individualized care and support, healthcare providers can help patients navigate the complexities of IC/BPS and achieve improved symptom control and overall well-being.

Quality of Life and Functional Outcomes in Interstitial Cystitis/Bladder Pain Syndrome (IC/BPS)

Interstitial Cystitis/Bladder Pain Syndrome (IC/BPS) significantly impacts patients' quality of life (QoL) and functional outcomes. Understanding and improving these aspects are essential for comprehensive management and enhancing overall well-being. This section explores the ways IC/ BPS affects quality of life and functional outcomes, methods for assessing these impacts, and strategies to improve them.

Impact of IC/BPS on Quality of Life

Physical Impact:

- **Chronic Pain:** IC/BPS is often characterized by persistent pelvic pain and discomfort, which can severely affect daily activities. The pain may be intermittent or constant, and its intensity can fluctuate, impacting patients' ability to perform routine tasks and engage in social activities.

- **Urinary Symptoms:** Frequent and urgent urination, along with nocturia (nighttime urination), can disrupt daily routines and sleep patterns. These symptoms often lead to fatigue, decreased physical activity, and reduced overall vitality.

- **Sexual Dysfunction:** Many patients with IC/BPS experience sexual dysfunction, including pain during intercourse and decreased libido. This can affect intimate relationships and contribute to emotional and psychological stress.

Emotional and Psychological Impact:

- **Mental Health Issues:** The chronic nature of IC/BPS and its associated symptoms can lead to anxiety, depression, and emotional distress. Patients often face challenges coping with the unpredictability and severity of their condition.

- **Social Isolation:** Due to symptoms such as frequent urination and pain, patients may withdraw from social activities and relationships. This social isolation can exacerbate feelings of loneliness and impact mental well-being.

- **Coping Strategies:** Effective coping strategies, including psychological support and cognitive-behavioral therapy (CBT), can help patients manage the emotional impact of IC/BPS. Patient education and support groups can also provide valuable resources for coping and resilience.

Functional Limitations:

- **Daily Functioning:** IC/BPS symptoms can limit patients' ability to engage in daily activities such as work, household chores, and recreational activities. The need for frequent restroom breaks and the discomfort associated with the condition can reduce productivity and participation in life activities.

- **Work Impairment:** For many patients, IC/BPS affects work performance and attendance. The need to manage symptoms and frequent urination can lead to absenteeism and decreased job satisfaction.

- **Physical Activity:** Pain and discomfort may limit physical activity and exercise, contributing to deconditioning and impacting overall health. Regular exercise is important for managing symptoms and maintaining physical health, but it may be challenging for patients with severe symptoms.

Methods for Assessing Quality of Life and Functional Outcomes

Patient-Reported Outcome Measures (PROMs):

- **Symptom Questionnaires:** Tools such as the Interstitial Cystitis Symptom Index (ICSI) and the O'Leary-Sant Questionnaire are commonly used to assess symptom severity and impact on daily life. These questionnaires help quantify the frequency, intensity, and effects of IC/BPS symptoms.

- **Quality of Life Scales:** Instruments like the Short Form 36 (SF-36) and the Patient-Reported Outcomes Measurement Information System (PROMIS) are used to evaluate overall health-related quality of life. These scales assess various domains, including physical functioning, emotional well-being, and social functioning.

- **Pain Scales:** The Visual Analog Scale (VAS) and the Brief Pain Inventory (BPI) are used to measure pain intensity and its impact on daily life. These scales help in understanding the extent of pain and its effect on quality of life.

Functional Assessments:

- **Bladder Diaries:** Keeping a bladder diary allows patients to track urinary frequency, urgency, and fluid intake. This information helps healthcare providers understand symptom patterns and make informed treatment decisions.

- **Urodynamic Studies:** Urodynamics assess bladder function, capacity, and detrusor activity. These studies provide objective data on bladder performance and can help evaluate the impact of IC/BPS on bladder function.

- **Functional Performance Measures:** Tools to assess physical performance, such as the 6-Minute Walk Test (6MWT), can help evaluate physical endurance and functional capacity. These measures can provide insights into how IC/BPS affects physical activity levels.

Strategies to Improve Quality of Life and Functional Outcomes

Treatment and Symptom Management:

- **Comprehensive Treatment Plans:** A multifaceted approach to treatment, including pharmacological, non-pharmacological, and interventional therapies, can help manage symptoms and improve quality of life. Tailoring treatment plans to individual needs and regularly adjusting them based on response is essential.

- **Multidisciplinary Care:** Coordinated care involving urologists, pain specialists, physical therapists, dietitians, and mental health professionals ensures that all aspects of the condition are addressed. This holistic approach can improve symptom control and enhance overall well-being.

Patient Education and Self-Management:

- **Education Programs:** Providing patients with information about IC/BPS, symptom management, and self-care strategies can empower them to manage their condition more effectively. Education should include guidance on bladder training, dietary modifications, and pain management techniques.

- **Self-Management Skills:** Teaching patients self-management skills, such as stress reduction techniques and coping strategies, can help them handle the emotional and psychological aspects of IC/BPS. Mindfulness, relaxation exercises, and cognitive-behavioral techniques can be beneficial.

Support and Counseling:

- **Support Groups:** Connecting patients with support groups and peer networks can provide emotional support and practical advice. Sharing experiences with others who have IC/BPS can help patients feel less isolated and more understood.

- **Counseling Services:** Access to mental health counseling and therapy can address psychological issues related to IC/BPS, such as anxiety and depression. Counseling can provide coping strategies, emotional support, and help patients navigate the challenges of living with a chronic condition.

Lifestyle Modifications:

- **Diet and Nutrition:** Dietary modifications, such as

avoiding bladder irritants and following a bladder-friendly diet, can help reduce symptoms and improve quality of life. Nutritional counseling can assist patients in making health-conscious choices.

- **Physical Activity:** Encouraging regular physical activity within the limits of the patient's symptoms can improve physical fitness, reduce stress, and enhance overall health. Exercise programs should be tailored to individual capabilities and symptom levels.

Long-Term Monitoring and Follow-Up:

- **Regular Assessments:** Ongoing monitoring of symptoms, functional outcomes, and quality of life through regular follow-up visits ensures that treatment plans remain effective and adjusted as needed.

- **Patient Feedback:** Regular feedback from patients about their experiences and challenges helps healthcare providers make informed decisions about treatment and support strategies.

Conclusion

Quality of life and functional outcomes are profoundly affected by Interstitial Cystitis/Bladder Pain Syndrome (IC/BPS), impacting various aspects of patients' physical, emotional, and social well-being. Assessing these impacts through patient-reported outcome measures and functional assessments provides valuable insights into the condition's effects. Effective management involves a combination of comprehensive treatment, patient education, self-management strategies, and support services. By addressing these aspects holistically and coordinating care, healthcare providers can improve the overall quality of life and functional outcomes for patients with IC/BPS, helping them lead fulfilling and manageable lives despite their chronic condition.

CHAPTER 7: HOLISTIC AND INTEGRATIVE APPROACHES

Lifestyle Modifications for Interstitial Cystitis/Bladder Pain Syndrome (IC/BPS)

Lifestyle modifications are a critical component in managing Interstitial Cystitis/Bladder Pain Syndrome (IC/BPS). They can help mitigate symptoms, improve overall well-being, and enhance the effectiveness of other treatments. This section delves into two crucial lifestyle modifications: exercise and physical activity, and sleep hygiene. Each of these factors plays a significant role in the management of IC/BPS and can contribute to better health outcomes.

Exercise and Physical Activity

The Role of Exercise in IC/BPS Management:

Exercise and physical activity can have a profound impact on managing IC/BPS. Regular physical activity helps regulate various bodily functions and can alleviate many of the symptoms associated with IC/BPS, including pain, urinary frequency, and overall discomfort.

Benefits of Exercise for IC/BPS Patients:

Pain Management:

Exercise promotes the release of endorphins, the body's natural painkillers, which can help reduce the perception of pain. For IC/BPS patients, regular physical activity may help manage pelvic pain and discomfort.

- **Application:** Engaging in low-impact exercises such as walking, swimming, or cycling can provide pain relief without exacerbating symptoms. Gentle stretching and yoga can also help alleviate muscle tension and pain in the pelvic region.

- **Scientific Basis:** Endorphins released during exercise interact with opioid receptors in the brain, reducing the perception of pain and improving mood. Additionally, regular exercise can help modulate the body's stress response, which may further alleviate pain.

Improved Bladder Function:

Regular physical activity can help improve bladder function by strengthening the muscles of the pelvic floor and enhancing overall bladder control. Exercise can also help reduce urinary frequency and urgency.

- **Application:** Pelvic floor exercises, such as Kegel exercises, can strengthen the muscles that support the bladder and improve bladder control. Incorporating these exercises into a regular fitness routine can benefit IC/BPS patients.

- **Scientific Basis:** Strengthening the pelvic floor muscles can enhance support for the bladder, potentially improving bladder capacity and control. This can reduce symptoms of urgency and frequency.

Enhanced Mood and Stress Reduction:

Exercise has well-documented benefits for mental health, including reducing symptoms of anxiety and depression. For IC/BPS patients, managing stress and improving mood can have a positive impact on symptom severity.

- **Application:** Activities such as aerobic exercises, strength training, and recreational sports can enhance mood and reduce stress. Finding enjoyable activities can also contribute to consistent participation in exercise.

- **Scientific Basis:** Exercise increases the production of neurotransmitters like serotonin and dopamine, which are associated with improved mood and reduced anxiety. Regular physical activity helps regulate the stress response, potentially alleviating stress-related symptoms.

Types of Exercise Suitable for IC/BPS Patients:

Low-Impact Aerobic Exercises:

Low-impact aerobic exercises are well-suited for IC/BPS patients as they provide cardiovascular benefits without placing excessive strain on the body.

- **Examples:** Walking, swimming, and cycling are ideal choices. These activities can be adjusted in intensity and duration based on individual comfort levels.

- **Benefits:** These exercises help improve cardiovascular health, enhance endurance, and contribute to overall physical fitness without exacerbating IC/BPS symptoms.

Pelvic Floor Exercises:

Pelvic floor exercises, including Kegel exercises, focus on strengthening the muscles that support the bladder and pelvic organs.

- **Application:** Patients can perform Kegel exercises by contracting and relaxing the muscles used to stop the flow of urine. These exercises can be done multiple times a day and incorporated into daily routines.

- **Benefits:** Strengthening the pelvic floor muscles can improve bladder control, reduce symptoms of urgency and frequency, and enhance overall pelvic health.

Stretching and Yoga:

Stretching and yoga are beneficial for improving flexibility, reducing muscle tension, and promoting relaxation.

- **Application:** Gentle stretching and yoga poses can help alleviate pelvic muscle tension and improve overall physical comfort. Yoga practices focused on breath control and relaxation can also support stress management.

- **Benefits:** Stretching and yoga can enhance flexibility, reduce muscle tightness, and promote relaxation, which can help alleviate IC/BPS symptoms and improve overall well-being.

Guidelines for Incorporating Exercise into Daily Life:

Starting Slowly:

Patients should begin with low-intensity exercises and gradually increase the intensity as tolerated. It is important to listen to the body and avoid overexertion.

- **Application:** Start with short sessions of low-impact activities and gradually build up duration and intensity. Monitoring symptoms and adjusting exercise routines as needed is essential.

Setting Realistic Goals:

Setting achievable and realistic exercise goals can help maintain motivation and track progress.

- **Application:** Establish specific, measurable goals for exercise frequency, duration, and type. Regularly reassess and adjust goals based on progress and symptom changes.

Seeking Professional Guidance:

Working with a physical therapist or fitness professional can provide personalized recommendations and ensure that exercises are performed correctly.

- **Application:** A physical therapist specializing in pelvic health can offer guidance on appropriate exercises and techniques for managing IC/BPS symptoms. They can also provide modifications based on individual needs.

Sleep Hygiene

The Importance of Sleep for IC/BPS Patients:

Adequate and restful sleep is essential for overall health and well-being. For IC/BPS patients, poor sleep quality can exacerbate symptoms, including pain and urinary frequency. Effective sleep hygiene practices can improve sleep quality and contribute to better symptom management.

Factors Affecting Sleep in IC/BPS:

Nocturia:

Frequent nighttime urination (nocturia) is a common symptom of IC/BPS that can disrupt sleep and lead to sleep deprivation.

- **Application:** Managing nocturia through lifestyle modifications, such as fluid restriction before bedtime and bladder training, can help reduce nighttime awakenings and improve sleep quality.

Pain and Discomfort:

Chronic pain and discomfort associated with IC/BPS can interfere with the ability to fall asleep and stay asleep.

- **Application:** Pain management strategies, including medication, physical therapy, and relaxation techniques, can help alleviate discomfort and improve sleep quality.

Sleep Hygiene Practices:

Establishing a Consistent Sleep Schedule:

Maintaining a regular sleep schedule helps regulate the body's internal clock and promotes restful sleep.

- **Application:** Set a consistent bedtime and wake-up

time, even on weekends. Create a relaxing bedtime routine to signal to the body that it is time to wind down.

- **Benefits:** A consistent sleep schedule helps regulate circadian rhythms, making it easier to fall asleep and wake up feeling refreshed.

Creating a Comfortable Sleep Environment:

A sleep-conducive environment can enhance sleep quality by minimizing disturbances and promoting relaxation.

- **Application:** Ensure that the sleep environment is cool, dark, and quiet. Invest in a comfortable mattress and pillows, and remove electronic devices that may interfere with sleep.

- **Benefits:** A comfortable sleep environment supports relaxation and minimizes disruptions, contributing to better sleep quality.

Limiting Stimulants and Distractions:

Avoiding stimulants and distractions before bedtime can help prepare the body for restful sleep.

- **Application:** Limit caffeine and nicotine intake in the hours leading up to bedtime. Avoid heavy meals and vigorous exercise close to bedtime. Establish a relaxing pre-sleep routine, such as reading or taking a warm bath.

- **Benefits:** Reducing stimulants and distractions promotes relaxation and helps the body transition smoothly into sleep.

Managing Fluid Intake:

Managing fluid intake can help reduce nighttime awakenings due to frequent urination.

- **Application:** Limit fluid intake in the evening, particularly in the hours before bedtime. Avoid beverages that can irritate the bladder, such as caffeine and alcohol.

- **Benefits:** Reducing fluid intake before bedtime can help minimize nocturia and improve uninterrupted sleep.

Addressing Pain and Discomfort:

Implementing strategies to manage pain and discomfort can enhance sleep quality.

- **Application:** Use pain management techniques, such as relaxation exercises, physical therapy, or medication, to address discomfort before bedtime. Experiment with different sleeping positions to find the most comfortable one.

- **Benefits:** Effective pain management improves comfort and promotes restful sleep.

Additional Strategies for Better Sleep:

Cognitive Behavioral Therapy for Insomnia (CBT-I):

Cognitive Behavioral Therapy for Insomnia (CBT-I) is a structured program designed to address sleep difficulties by changing behaviors and thoughts related to sleep.

- **Application:** CBT-I typically involves working with a trained therapist to identify and address sleep-related issues. Techniques may include cognitive restructuring, sleep restriction, and behavioral interventions.

- **Benefits:** CBT-I can help address underlying sleep disorders, improve sleep quality, and enhance overall well-being.

Relaxation Techniques:

Incorporating relaxation techniques into the bedtime routine can help calm the mind and body.

- **Application:** Practice relaxation techniques such as deep breathing exercises, progressive muscle relaxation, or guided imagery before bedtime to promote relaxation and prepare for sleep.

- **Benefits:** Relaxation techniques can help reduce stress and anxiety, making it easier to fall asleep and stay asleep.

Conclusion

Lifestyle modifications, including exercise and physical activity and sleep hygiene, play a crucial role in managing Interstitial Cystitis/Bladder Pain Syndrome (IC/BPS). Regular physical activity can help manage pain, improve bladder function,

Integrative Therapies for Interstitial Cystitis/Bladder Pain Syndrome (IC/BPS)

Integrative therapies offer a holistic approach to managing Interstitial Cystitis/Bladder Pain Syndrome (IC/BPS) by combining conventional medical treatments with alternative and complementary practices. These therapies focus on the overall well-being of the patient, aiming to address not only the physical symptoms but also the emotional and psychological aspects of the condition. This section explores two prominent integrative therapies for IC/BPS: acupuncture and traditional Chinese medicine, and herbal medicine and nutraceuticals.

Acupuncture and Traditional Chinese Medicine (TCM)

Overview of Acupuncture and TCM:

Acupuncture is a key component of Traditional Chinese Medicine (TCM), which has been practiced for thousands of years. It involves the insertion of fine needles into specific points on the body to stimulate energy flow (Qi) and restore balance. TCM encompasses a broader range of practices, including herbal medicine, dietary recommendations, and qi gong.

Mechanisms of Acupuncture:

Qi and Meridians:

In TCM, the body is thought to have pathways called meridians through which Qi (vital energy) flows. Blockages or imbalances in Qi flow are believed to contribute to pain and disease.

- **Application:** Acupuncture aims to restore the proper flow of Qi by inserting needles into specific acupuncture points along the meridians. This practice is intended to balance the body's energy, alleviate pain, and promote healing.

- **Scientific Basis:** Acupuncture points correspond to specific areas that are thought to influence the flow of Qi. Stimulation of these points is believed to modulate various physiological processes, including pain perception and inflammation.

Neurotransmitter and Endorphin Release:

Acupuncture has been shown to influence the release of neurotransmitters and endorphins, which play a role in pain modulation and mood regulation.

- **Application:** Acupuncture needles are thought to stimulate the release of endorphins, the body's natural painkillers, and neurotransmitters that can help reduce pain and promote a sense of well-being.

- **Scientific Basis:** Research suggests that acupuncture may enhance the release of endorphins and modulate neurotransmitter systems involved in pain perception and emotional regulation.

Evidence of Acupuncture for IC/BPS:

Clinical Studies and Outcomes:

Several studies have investigated the efficacy of acupuncture for managing IC/BPS symptoms. Results have been mixed, but some evidence suggests that acupuncture may help alleviate pain and improve quality of life.

- **Application:** Clinical trials have shown that acupuncture can reduce pelvic pain, urinary frequency, and urgency in some IC/BPS patients. Acupuncture treatment plans typically involve multiple sessions over a period of weeks or months.

- **Scientific Basis:** Studies have demonstrated that acupuncture can lead to significant improvements in symptoms for some patients. However, results can vary based on individual factors, including the severity of symptoms and the specific acupuncture points used.

Safety and Considerations:

Acupuncture is generally considered safe when performed by a qualified practitioner. However, it is essential to ensure that needles are sterile and that the practitioner is trained in proper techniques.

- **Application:** Patients should seek licensed acupuncturists who adhere to established safety standards. It is also important to discuss acupuncture as part of a comprehensive treatment plan with their healthcare provider.

- **Scientific Basis:** Adherence to safety protocols and practitioner qualifications is crucial for minimizing risks and maximizing the therapeutic benefits of acupuncture.

Traditional Chinese Medicine (TCM) in IC/BPS:

Herbal Medicine:

TCM also includes the use of herbal remedies to address various health conditions. Herbal formulas are tailored to individual needs based on TCM principles.

- **Application:** Herbal remedies for IC/BPS may include ingredients known for their anti-inflammatory, analgesic, or diuretic properties. Formulas are customized based on the patient's specific symptoms and overall health.

- **Scientific Basis:** Herbal medicine in TCM is often used to complement acupuncture and other treatments. Evidence for specific herbs and formulas can vary, and patients should consult with knowledgeable practitioners.

Dietary Recommendations:

Dietary guidelines in TCM focus on balancing the body's internal environment through food choices and eating habits.

- **Application:** Patients may receive dietary advice to avoid foods that are believed to exacerbate symptoms, such as spicy or acidic foods. Emphasis is placed on incorporating foods that promote healing and balance.

- **Scientific Basis:** TCM dietary recommendations are based on principles of balancing energy and supporting overall health. While scientific evidence may be limited, dietary modifications can contribute to symptom management.

Qi Gong and Tai Chi:

Qi Gong and Tai Chi are mind-body practices that involve slow, deliberate movements and breathing exercises to promote Qi flow and overall health.

- **Application:** These practices can be incorporated into a daily routine to enhance physical fitness, reduce stress, and support overall well-being. They can complement other treatments and improve quality of life.

- **Scientific Basis:** Research suggests that Qi Gong and Tai Chi can improve physical function, reduce pain, and enhance mental health, making them valuable complementary therapies for IC/BPS patients.

Herbal Medicine and Nutraceuticals

Overview of Herbal Medicine and Nutraceuticals:

Herbal medicine and nutraceuticals involve the use of plant-based compounds and dietary supplements to support health and manage symptoms. These approaches can be integrated into the treatment plan for IC/BPS to provide additional symptom relief and improve overall health.

Herbal Medicine for IC/BPS:

Commonly Used Herbs:

Several herbs have been traditionally used in the management of urinary and pelvic conditions. Some of these include:

- **Marshmallow Root (Althaea officinalis):** Known for its soothing properties, marshmallow root is used to alleviate bladder irritation and inflammation.

- **Slippery Elm (Ulmus rubra):** Contains mucilage, which may help protect and soothe the bladder lining.

- **Cranberry (Vaccinium macrocarpon):** Often used for urinary tract health, cranberry is thought to have anti-inflammatory and antibacterial properties.

- **Dandelion (Taraxacum officinale):** Known for its diuretic properties, dandelion may help with urinary frequency and bladder health.

- **Uva Ursi (Arctostaphylos uva-ursi):** Traditionally used for its astringent and antimicrobial effects, which may support urinary tract health.

Evidence and Efficacy:

While some herbal remedies have historical use and anecdotal support, scientific evidence on their efficacy for IC/BPS can vary.

- **Application:** Herbal treatments should be considered as complementary options and used with caution. Consulting with a healthcare provider knowledgeable in herbal medicine is essential for safe and effective use.

- **Scientific Basis:** Research on individual herbs may provide insight into their potential benefits. However, more rigorous clinical trials are needed to establish definitive efficacy and safety for IC/BPS.

Safety Considerations:

Herbal remedies can interact with prescription medications and may cause side effects. It is important to use herbs under the guidance of a qualified healthcare provider.

- **Application:** Patients should disclose all herbal supplements and medications to their healthcare provider to avoid potential interactions and ensure safe use.

- **Scientific Basis:** Some herbs may have contraindications or adverse effects. Ensuring that herbs are used appropriately and safely is crucial for patient safety.

Nutraceuticals for IC/BPS:

Key Nutraceuticals:

Nutraceuticals are dietary supplements that provide health benefits beyond basic nutrition. For IC/BPS, certain nutraceuticals may be considered:

- **L-Arginine:** An amino acid that may support nitric oxide production and improve blood flow, potentially benefiting bladder function.

- **Omega-3 Fatty Acids:** Found in fish oil, omega-3s have anti-inflammatory properties that may help reduce inflammation and pain associated with IC/BPS.

- **Quercetin:** A flavonoid with antioxidant and anti-inflammatory properties, which may help manage symptoms of IC/BPS.

- **Vitamin D:** Supports immune function and may have anti-inflammatory effects, potentially benefiting bladder health.
- **Probiotics:** Support gut health and may contribute to overall immune function, which can be relevant for managing IC/BPS symptoms.

Evidence and Research:

Research on nutraceuticals often focuses on their general health benefits rather than specific effects on IC/BPS. Evidence for their use in IC/BPS may be preliminary and require further investigation.

- **Application:** Nutraceuticals should be used as part of a comprehensive treatment plan, with careful consideration of their potential benefits and risks.
- **Scientific Basis:** Some nutraceuticals have shown promise in preliminary studies, but more research is needed to confirm their efficacy and safety for IC/BPS management.

Safety and Dosage:

Proper dosage and safety are critical when using nutraceuticals. Consulting with a healthcare provider ensures appropriate use and avoids potential interactions.

- **Application:** Follow recommended dosages and consult with a healthcare provider before starting any new supplements, especially if combining them with other treatments.
- **Scientific Basis:** Adherence to dosage guidelines and awareness of potential interactions are important for the safe and effective use of nutraceuticals.

Made in the USA
Coppell, TX
12 November 2024

40091745R00095